DR. BUYNAK'S

1-2-3

DIABETES DIET

Robert J. Buynak, MD

with Gregory L. Guthrie

D1125670

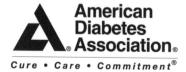

American
Diabetes
Association.
Cure • Care • Commitment®

Director, Book Publishing, John Fedor; *Managing Editor, Book Publishing,* Abe Ogden; *Editor,* Abe Ogden, Greg Guthrie; *Production Manager,* Melissa Sprott; *Composition,* Melissa Sprott; *Cover Design,* Koncept, Inc.; *Printer,* United Graphics, Incorporated.

Printed in the United States of America
1 3 5 7 9 10 8 6 4 2

The suggestions and information contained in this publication are generally consistent with the *Clinical Practice Recommendations* and other policies of the American Diabetes Association, but they do not represent the policy or position of the Association or any of its boards or committees. Reasonable steps have been taken to ensure the accuracy of the information presented. However, the American Diabetes Association cannot ensure the safety or efficacy of any product or service described in this publication. Individuals are advised to consult a physician or other appropriate health care professional before undertaking any diet or exercise program or taking any medication referred to in this publication. Professionals must use and apply their own professional judgment, experience, and training and should not rely solely on the information contained in this publication before prescribing any diet, exercise, or medication. The American Diabetes Association—its officers, directors, employees, volunteers, and members—assumes no responsibility or liability for personal or other injury, loss, or damage that may result from the suggestions or information in this publication.

⊗ The paper in this publication meets the requirements of the ANSI Standard Z39.48-1992 (permanence of paper).

ADA titles may be purchased for business or promotional use or for special sales. To purchase this book in large quantities, or for custom editions of this book with your logo, contact Lee Romano Sequeira, Special Sales & Promotions, at the address below, or at LRomano@diabetes.org or 703-299-2046.

American Diabetes Association
1701 North Beauregard Street
Alexandria, Virginia 22311

Library of Congress Cataloging-in-Publication Data
Buynak, Robert.
    Dr. Buynak's 1-2-3 diabetes diet : a step-by-step approach to weight loss without gimmicks or risks / Robert Buynak with Gregory L. Guthrie.
        p. cm.
    Includes bibliographical references and index.
    ISBN 1-58040-243-7 (alk. paper)
        1. Diabetes—Diet therapy. 2. Diabetes—Nutritional aspects.
    I. Guthrie, Gregory L. II. Title. III. Title: 1-2-3 diabetes diet. IV. Title: One-two-three diabetes diet.
    RC662.B89 2006
    616.4'620654--dc22
                                                2005035337

Contents

Acknowledgments

I owe many thanks to those who had a hand in the writing of this book. I owe special thanks to Abe Ogden of the American Diabetes Association for making this project become a reality and to Greg Guthrie for his hard work in editing the manuscript. In addition, my appreciation goes out to the multiple reviewers of the book for their insights and suggestions.

To my patients with diabetes and the staff at Hilltop Community Health Center, thank you for your daily inspiration—may we find good health together. To Michelle, Shanna, and Darla, thanks for keeping the office going. Finally, to my children and family and especially my wife, Melissa, thanks for your support and for encouraging us to eat our vegetables.

Introduction

Talk of diabetes is everywhere these days—on the news, in magazines, around the table during the holidays. After all, a lot Americans have diabetes. You or a loved one probably has diabetes (why else would you be reading a diabetes diet book?). Maybe you've struggled with the disease for many years. Like many people with this disease, you may also be feeling a lot of pressure to take care of your blood sugar and watch your diet. And like most, you may be feeling that the disease has taken over your life.

My medical practice, like that of most doctors, is full of people who have diabetes and are overweight or obese. I practice in an industrial Midwestern community and find myself constantly facing the same type of patients: adults struggling with their weight and at risk for or already diagnosed with type 2 diabetes. Nearly all of these people are hard-working Americans who have fallen into bad habits. And almost all want to lead healthier lives but don't know where to begin. Fortunately, the path to better health is easier to follow than many believe.

Diabetes and diet go hand in hand. As most doctors will tell you, there is one thing standing between people with diabetes and good health: the American lifestyle. We eat too much food, often eat the wrong types of food, and lead very inactive lifestyles. Even those who work on their feet don't get enough aerobic exercise and often don't make good food choices. As a result, obesity and diabetes are the new American epidemics. If America is going to conquer these epidemics, we have to try to understand the relationship between diabetes and diet and find ways we can change our approach to health.

My experience with people with diabetes and my own life experiences have taught me much about the average lifestyle. To change this unhealthy routine and halt the spread of diabetes and obesity, people need two things: clear education and long-term motivation. The first part, education, isn't as hard as many people believe. I feel that most people actually know what food choices to make (see the box "Nutrition Confusion?"). The difficult part is changing our eating behaviors and changing those behaviors to last a lifetime. It is with these thoughts in mind that I have written this book.

Nutrition Confusion?

Many of my patients claim that they are confused about nutrition. You may feel the same way, and this is understandable. One day, carbohydrates are the foundations of a healthy diet; the next, they're the reason everyone's so overweight. One report says that eggs are a health food, while another says they contribute to heart disease.

There are a few reasons for this conflicting information. First, nutrition research is not a clear-cut process, and the results should not be treated as gospel. Many times, news organizations and health magazines will pick and choose information from small, short-term—and sometimes unreliable—studies and present it as scientific fact. This can be very misleading. Sometimes these studies simply find information that suggests more serious research is needed or that there are occasional exceptions to the rule. Sometimes studies are just not conducted properly. This is often not mentioned on the nightly news or in magazines, industries where ratings and readership are sometimes more important than your best interests.

And let's not forget another culprit—ourselves. Americans have become selective students of nutrition and will often use nutrition news to rationalize making decisions we know are not healthy. When we hear on the news that a high-fat diet is just fine, we use this as an excuse to eat plates full of bacon (and ignore the rest of the diet that suggests staying away from starches). But when we hear about research that proves fruits and vegetables are still good for us, we ignore it and chalk it up to the fact that "the experts are always changing their minds." Be honest with yourself: you know what selections are not healthy. And even those foods that *are* healthy still need to be eaten in moderation.

Nutrition information can be confusing. There's nothing wrong with having questions. Hopefully, I'll answer many of them in this book. But I have enough faith in my patients and in you to believe we can all make the right choices.

In this book, I have tried to simplify the guidelines that help people with diabetes lead healthy lives and gain control of their weight and blood sugar. I have reduced the process to a three-step approach. I also have avoided pyramids, graphs, and other popular meal-planning tools because I feel we've all seen them and we've all chosen not to use them. Instead, I have focused on counting numbers. Counting is something everyone can do, and I have found with my patients that this is the most effective approach to losing weight.

Like I said before, most people actually know what it takes to follow a healthy diet. The challenge is in encouraging and motivating people to follow through on what they already know. I know you are motivated to improve your health or you wouldn't have read this far. Now it's time to put that motivation to work.

First Things First:

What You Need to Know about Diabetes and Weight Loss

Chapter 1
Diabetes by the Numbers

I'm going to get straight to the point. Twenty-one million Americans have diabetes. Almost 60% of Americans—127 million people—are overweight, obese, or severely obese. Two out of three people diagnosed with type 2 diabetes are overweight or obese.

These numbers and statistics may be new to you or you may have heard them before. Maybe they're frightening to you. Maybe they don't have any impact at all. Health care officials often toss out these large figures imagining they will scare the entire population into taking care of themselves. It never seems to work. Instead, these huge numbers are hard to visualize, fail to make any kind of impact, and sometimes make people more resistant to making healthy lifestyle changes. If there are so many overweight people with diabetes, it must not be that big of a deal, right?

Q&A
Am I a "diabetic" or a "person with diabetes"?
This question may not seem important, but it actually underlines a very critical attitude toward diabetes. People with diabetes have no problem calling themselves "diabetic." But do people with cancer call themselves "cancerous"? People have asthma, but they don't walk around calling themselves "asthmatics." Why is diabetes different? In some ways, this shows how resigned people are to their situation and how little they regard the danger of diabetes. So let's drop the "diabetic" tag. You may have diabetes, but it doesn't define you and it's not an excuse to give up on taking care of yourself.

Finally, a Diet for People with Diabetes

Not quite. When I use the word "diet" throughout this book, I mean it in terms of what you normally eat. When most people hear the word *diet,* they think of starving themselves, losing a little weight, and then putting it back on after they're off that "diet." That's not what I mean. Following a healthy diet doesn't have a time line; it should last throughout your entire life.

More importantly, there is no one specific diet that people with diabetes should follow. The old rule of a "diabetic diet" is outdated. It used to be "no sugar, no candy, and no doughnuts unless you're low," but we've been trying to get away from this for years. That "diabetic diet" simply doesn't help people who are trying to control their blood sugar. Still, I hear people talk about how people with diabetes shouldn't ever eat sugar—*ever*. This is simply untrue. Here's the secret about how people with diabetes should eat: *If you have diabetes, you need to eat healthy.* Period. I'll say it again: if you have diabetes, your diet is a healthy meal plan that's good for anyone. The main difference will be in how much attention you have to pay to the carbohydrate content of your foods and how these foods affect your blood glucose levels.

Instead, let's focus on number one—you. Regardless of whether you believe that there is an epidemic of obesity and/or diabetes, the straight facts show that if you have type 2 diabetes, you are at risk for developing multiple medical problems and you need to take care of this dangerous situation. The most important aspect of this equation is you.

WHY "1-2-3?"

I've named my diet the 1-2-3 Diabetes Diet for a few reasons. First, this approach to meal planning is loosely based on three, easy-to-understand steps. I also really like the method of using numbers and counting. Many people are uneasy about numbers (blame high school algebra), but I have found that compared to the graphs and charts and pyramids often used in meal plans, numbers are actually easier to understand. Also, many of the things related to caring for your diabetes will come to you in the form of numbers. What's your blood sugar level? What's your A1C? What's your blood pressure? If you have diabetes, you should be very aware of the role numbers have in your life. Finally, I feel that the simple, no-nonsense approach described in this book is as easy as 1-2-3. There are no tricks or gimmicks. You just need a little bit of dedication, hard work, and common sense. I'd bet we can all scratch that together if it means that we could live a little longer and a little healthier.

The 1-2-3 Diabetes Diet

Following are the 1-2-3 steps of the Diabetes Diet you can follow for weight loss and better health:

1. Think about your eating habits.

2. Make healthy changes.
3. Stick with it.

Sounds simple, doesn't it? Naturally, we'll discuss each step in much more detail later in the book. But for the most part, these are the basics of my plan for losing weight.

If you've flipped through this book, you may have realized that the 1-2-3 Diabetes Diet is not going to tell you exactly what to eat every day for the rest of your life. Those types of diets are simply too rigid and do not work in the long run. Instead, I'm going to provide you with the tools you need to build healthy habits that will last a lifetime. No two people are exactly alike, so why should everyone have to eat the same thing?

Chapter 2
Weighty Issues:
Scales Don't Lie

Many people don't consider a few extra pounds that big of a deal. They claim they're comfortable with their bodies and don't need to live up to any unrealistic ideal spread by the media. They are happy with themselves and don't feel the need to change. And you know what? I think there's a lot of good in this attitude. Everyone should feel happy with who they are.

However, there is more involved with being overweight than self-image. Carrying around a few extra pounds may not always be a problem. You don't need to look like a swimsuit model or have defined abs. That is a little unrealistic, especially as we get older. You do need to be healthy, though, and when those "few" extra pounds are actually 30 or 40 extra pounds, you're putting yourself at serious risk for a variety of health problems. This is no longer a matter of vanity; it's a matter of damaging your body.

In the off chance that you don't believe that obesity or being overweight is a problem, think about this. Obesity is becoming an American epidemic, and it is nearly impossible to talk about type 2 diabetes without also considering a person's weight. A greater and greater percentage of Americans are overweight or obese with every passing year. The reasons for this obesity epidemic are complex, but too much food and not enough exercise are at least partly to blame. Being overweight or obese is something we can control, and considering that being overweight carries so many dangerous health risks, we should all take the effort to shed those few extra pounds.

Sedentary Lifestyle

You've probably heard this term before, but may not know what it means exactly. A sedentary lifestyle is one that involves a lot of sitting and, generally, little activity or movement. Because the majority of the work we do in America these days takes place in offices and on computers, the lack of physical activity makes us more likely to gain weight. This is because we're not burning many of the calories we consume over the course of a normal workday. We also spend many hours during the day in the car, which isn't a particularly physical activity. Our towns and suburbs are built for driving, not walking. Our leisure activities involve sitting around the television, surfing the Internet, and playing video games. Suddenly, you can see why overweight and obesity are increasingly common among Americans. Some of you out there still work physical jobs (such as construction, moving jobs, etc.), but the problem these days is that our American diet provides so many calories that it far surpasses any amount that we could burn while working or during leisure activities. This, in a nutshell, is the sedentary lifestyle.

The Vital Connection: Obesity and Your Health

If you develop type 2 diabetes, carrying around those extra pounds isn't anything you can just shrug off anymore. It is a real problem. If you are overweight and have diabetes, you must do something to address this common health issue. Here's why.

1. Obesity and overweight are risk factors for diabetes complications. If you have diabetes, being overweight or obese will increase the chances that you will develop dangerous diabetes complications, such as blindness, heart attack, or kidney disease. Losing weight will improve your chances of living a longer, healthier life—even if you do have diabetes.

2. Scientists have found that maintaining a healthy body weight is one of the most effective ways to control diabetes. The influence of obesity and overweight on the development of diabetes is reversible in the early stages of the disease. Diet and weight loss are often the first treatments for people with early type 2 diabetes (or pre-diabetes) because they are amazingly effective and relatively easy to accomplish.

3. Type 2 diabetes isn't the only health risk associated with being overweight. Overweight or obese people are at a higher risk of having high blood pressure, heart disease, and some cancers. Your weight is also connected with many other health problems. By losing weight, you can reduce your risk of encountering many of these problems.

Small Steps

If you want to improve your health through weight loss, you can start small. Just losing a little weight has a noticeable effect on your diabetes care. In the beginning, aim for modest weight loss. People who lose just 5% to 7% of their total body weight and maintain an exercise program normally see an improvement in their health. Here's what this means, and it can be done on a simple calculator. Let's say you weigh 240 pounds.

$240 \times 0.05 = 12$ pounds
$240 \times 0.07 = 17$ pounds

This is the formula:
[Your weight] $\times$ [0.05 or 0.07] = Initial Weight Loss Goal

Now it's time to find out what **your** initial weight-loss goal should be:

5% weight loss: (your weight) _____ $\times$ 0.05 = _____ pounds

7% weight loss: (your weight) _____ $\times$ 0.07 = _____ pounds

The thought of losing 12–17 pounds shouldn't be intimidating, especially because you should aim to lose about one pound a week. Use this limit as a starting point for the 1-2-3 Diabetes Diet. It may be better for you to lose more weight, but you should start with

Body Mass Index Table

BMI / Height (inches)	19	20	21	22	23	24	25	26	27	28	29	30	31	32	33	34	35
							Body Weight (pounds)										
58	91	96	100	105	110	115	119	124	129	134	138	143	148	153	158	162	167
59	94	99	104	109	114	119	124	128	133	138	143	148	153	158	163	168	173
60	97	102	107	112	118	123	128	133	138	143	148	153	158	163	168	174	179
61	100	106	111	116	122	127	132	137	143	148	153	158	164	169	174	180	185
62	104	109	115	120	126	131	136	142	147	153	158	164	169	175	180	186	191
63	107	113	118	124	130	135	141	146	152	158	163	169	175	180	186	191	197
64	110	116	122	128	134	140	145	151	157	163	169	174	180	186	192	197	204
65	114	120	126	132	138	144	150	156	162	168	174	180	186	192	198	204	210
66	118	124	130	136	142	148	155	161	167	173	179	186	192	198	204	210	216
67	121	127	134	140	146	153	159	166	172	178	185	191	198	204	211	217	223
68	125	131	138	144	151	158	164	171	177	184	190	197	203	210	216	223	230
69	128	135	142	149	155	162	169	176	182	189	196	203	209	216	223	230	236
70	132	139	146	153	160	167	174	181	188	195	202	209	216	222	229	236	243
71	136	143	150	157	165	172	179	186	193	200	208	215	222	229	236	243	250
72	140	147	154	162	169	177	184	191	199	206	213	221	228	235	242	250	258
73	144	151	159	166	174	182	189	197	204	212	219	227	235	242	250	257	265
74	148	155	163	171	179	186	194	202	210	218	225	233	241	249	256	264	272
75	152	160	168	176	184	192	200	208	216	224	232	240	248	256	264	272	279
76	156	164	172	180	189	197	205	213	221	230	238	246	254	263	271	279	287

Body Weight (pounds)

BMI / Height (inches)	36	37	38	39	40	41	42	43	44	45	46	47	48	49	50	51	52	53	54
58	172	177	181	186	191	196	201	205	210	215	220	224	229	234	239	244	248	253	258
59	178	183	188	193	198	203	208	212	217	222	227	232	237	242	247	252	257	262	267
60	184	189	194	199	204	209	215	220	225	230	235	240	245	250	255	261	266	271	276
61	190	195	201	206	211	217	222	227	232	238	243	248	254	259	264	269	275	280	285
62	196	202	207	213	218	224	229	235	240	246	251	256	262	267	273	278	284	289	295
63	203	208	214	220	225	231	237	242	248	254	259	265	270	278	282	287	293	299	304
64	209	215	221	227	232	238	244	250	256	262	267	273	279	285	291	296	302	308	314
65	216	222	228	234	240	246	252	258	264	270	276	282	288	294	300	306	312	318	324
66	223	229	235	241	247	253	260	266	272	278	284	291	297	303	309	315	322	328	334
67	230	236	242	249	255	261	268	274	280	287	293	299	306	312	319	325	331	338	344
68	236	243	249	256	262	269	276	282	289	295	302	308	315	322	328	335	341	348	354
69	243	250	257	263	270	277	284	291	297	304	311	318	324	331	338	345	351	358	365
70	250	257	264	271	278	285	292	299	306	313	320	327	334	341	348	355	362	369	376
71	257	265	272	279	286	293	301	308	315	322	329	338	343	351	358	365	372	379	386
72	265	272	279	287	294	302	309	316	324	331	338	346	353	361	368	375	383	390	397
73	272	280	288	295	302	310	318	325	333	340	348	355	363	371	378	386	393	401	408
74	280	287	295	303	311	319	326	334	342	350	358	365	373	381	389	396	404	412	420
75	287	295	303	311	319	327	335	343	351	359	367	375	383	391	399	407	415	423	431
76	295	304	312	320	328	336	344	353	361	369	377	385	394	402	410	418	426	435	443

this. Small steps are a great beginning for any difficult and important task.

OKAY, WHERE'S THE SCALE?

When you're ready to begin your weight-loss program, you need to take some beginning steps to assess how much you weigh and where that extra weight is.

1. Know your body mass index. Your body mass index (also called BMI) assesses your body size in terms of height and weight. BMI is a pretty good indicator of how much total fat is in your body, but it's not very effective past that. We calculate BMI with a mathematical formula, and standardized charts show the results of those calculations. [See charts, pages 14–15.]

To find your current BMI, find the box for your height and read across until you reach the column that contains your weight. To find your ideal BMI, find the purple boxes that correspond to your height and match that to the corresponding weight. People with a BMI of 25 or greater are considered overweight, and those with a BMI of 30 or greater are obese.

Some Things to Consider about BMI

You may have already noticed or heard this, but looking at BMI is not a foolproof way to figure out how healthy you are. First off, BMI will not determine where you carry most of your fat, and research shows that carrying fat around your belly is more dangerous than carrying it in your hips and thighs. Second, BMI can't discern the difference between very muscular people (for example, athletes) and obese people. This is because muscle is more dense than fat, thus it weighs more. BMI only assesses your weight in relation to your height; it cannot determine whether you're fit or out of shape. BMI is only one tool out of many used to assess a person's body fat content. However, unless you're an Olympic athlete or a bodybuilder, your BMI will closely represent your overall body fat.

Additionally, the BMI charts are generic, meaning that they don't consider age or gender. For example, women typically have more body fat than men if they have the same BMI. Also, older people tend to lose more muscle mass as they age, so their BMI may underestimate the amount of total fat in their bodies.

---

2. Are you shaped like a pear or an apple? Did you know that being an apple shape (more fat around your middle), rather than a pear shape (more fat around your hips), puts you at greater risk for type 2 diabetes and heart disease? You can figure your shape by taking your waist circumference, which measures how far it is around your waist. There is some debate about this, but some research has suggested that waist circumference may be a better indicator of a person's risk of developing diabetes than BMI.

Here's how to figure out your waist circumference:
Just take a tape measure (a flexible, soft one is best) and place it snugly (but not tight) around your body at bellybutton height. This is your waist, despite where your pants may fit. Compare the length around your waist to the number below. If the length of your waist is the same or greater than the numbers below, you have too much weight around your waist.

Waist Circumference
Men: over 40 inches
Women: over 35 inches

3. Use the scale as a guide. Do you even have a scale? If not, you need to buy one. Many health professionals advise against using a scale while trying to lose weight. I disagree. Monitoring your weight is an excellent way to evaluate your progress and determine whether you need to make changes to your weight-loss plan. Keep in mind that there will be small fluctuations in your weight from day to day. Don't let this get you down. But if you find that you're consistently gaining weight over the course of a few weeks, then you should make changes. Similarly, if you're consistently losing weight over a week, keep at what you're doing. Try to weigh yourself every day, but at least three times a week. If it'll help motivate you, enter your weight on your food diary.

A scale serves as an impartial judge of how you are doing in your quest for better health. You can't argue with it, and negotiating with a scale is impossible. It will always tell you exactly how much you weigh.

Some people are understandably afraid to even step on a scale. If you're embarrassed by your weight, you may have avoided scales and avoided even knowing your weight. Just as in all parts of life, ignoring problems hardly makes them better. Not thinking about your weight and claiming ignorance may make you feel better about yourself for a little while, but it doesn't make the issue disappear. You can see it whenever you look in the mirror or try on clothes.

If you are going to lose weight and get healthy, you need to step on a scale. You need to face your fears and conquer them. Accept who you are and accept that that is you standing on the scale. It's not going to be that bad. Why? Because you're going to lose weight. In time, you'll begin to enjoy watching the progress you've made.

If I Can Stop Here for a Moment...

I'd like to congratulate you for making it this far. I know it doesn't seem like much—we're only a few pages in—but just getting to this point shows that you are motivated to lose weight, live healthier, and begin controlling your diabetes. This is not an easy process, but I promise you that the benefits will be worth every bit of effort you put into it. As we move forward through this book, keep in mind that motivation over the long term (the rest of your life!) is the key to being successful. There will be difficult times, but there will also be great times, such as getting your first good A1C test, buying clothes a size smaller, or just an overall sense of accomplishment.

I'll be spending the rest of this section talking about diabetes care and explaining things like A1C, and then it's on to the 1-2-3 Diabetes Diet. As you move forward, remember why you wanted to lose weight and be healthy in the first place and use that as motivation to keep you going.

Chapter 3
Type 2 Diabetes: What You Need to Know

This is primarily a diet book, so I'm not going to discuss the ins and outs of diabetes management and self-care at length. However, this is a diabetes diet book, so some discussion is necessary.

It is amazing how little some of my patients with diabetes know about the disease. Even those who have had diabetes for years confess to some puzzling misconceptions. For instance, during one memorable office visit, a patient who had been referred to me after an episode of diabetic ketoacidosis (DKA, a condition that results from very high blood glucose levels) told me she had stopped taking her diabetes medication. When I asked her why, she told me that food made her blood glucose go lower and the medication caused her blood glucose to go higher. She figured she would just eat food to keep her blood glucose low and stop messing with medications. To say the least, I was amazed; this woman had suffered from diabetes for years and obviously had no idea how the condition affected her body. I explained to her that food actually raises blood glucose and that diabetes medications lower the level of glucose in the blood, so she definitely needed to keep taking her medication or else she could expect more episodes of DKA. This completely surprised her. Apparently, no one had taken the time to explain to her exactly how diabetes works, and it could have led to some very dangerous results. This example is extreme, but misconceptions like this are not completely uncommon.

I relate this story here because it not only illustrates how confusing diabetes can be, but it also shows the importance of education when you're dealing with a disease that requires a lot of self-care. Diabetes is a chronic condition that needs to be treated day in and day out, which means the bulk of the responsibility falls on you, the person with diabetes. Because of this, you need to know as much about the disease, its complications, and its treatments as you can. With that in mind, this should not be the only diabetes book you own; there's simply too much you need to know. This is just the basics, but it should be a good start.

TYPE 2 DIABETES: A BRIEF EXPLANATION

Simply put, diabetes is any condition that results in high levels of glucose in a person's bloodstream. There are many ways this can happen, which is why there are different types of diabetes. Of the different types of diabetes there are three that are the most common—type 1 diabetes, type 2 diabetes, and gestational diabetes. Each of these conditions causes high blood glucose (or hyperglycemia), though the way they cause it is different, which I'll explain below. However, to understand how things can go wrong, you first need to understand how the body normally uses (or metabolizes) food when it is working properly.

Turning Food into Energy

For you to have the energy you need to walk, work, or keep your heart and lungs pumping, your body needs fuel. That fuel is food. Contained within the foods we eat is stored energy, which is measured in calories. When you check the label on a bag of potato chips and look at the number of calories, you're actually looking at how much energy is stored in a serving of those chips. Almost all of the calories, or energy, in food come from three nutrients—protein, fat, and carbohydrate. When you eat, your digestive system breaks down these nutrients and converts them into forms the body can use. Proteins help build and repair muscle and organ tissue. Fats help rebuild membranes in your cells and are stored as energy reserves. Any calories not used right away by your body are also stored away as fat. But for the pure energy used by cells to keep everything operating, your body prefers carbohydrate, which is converted to glucose during digestion.

The journey from undigested carbohydrate to glucose is a complex one. Basically, once you eat carbohydrate (and a few other nutrients, but mostly carb), the body converts it into glucose in the digestive system. This glucose is then released into the bloodstream so it can reach the cells that use it as fuel. However, and this is the important part for people with diabetes, glucose can't get into the cells on its own. For that, the body needs insulin. Insulin is a hormone produced in the pancreas, and it acts like a key that unlocks the door to the cells and allows glucose to enter. This glucose is then used by the cells to make energy. Without insulin, blood glucose remains in the bloodstream. When things are operating correctly, enough insulin is produced in the pancreas to meet the need created by the glucose levels in the blood. This insulin moves the glucose into cells and the cells use the glucose to fuel the activities that keep our bodies going.

Glucose can come from sources other than recently digested food as well. The liver stores glucose, which it releases periodically to ensure that the cells always have a source of energy. This occurs primarily when a person has not eaten for a while, something we call the *fasting state*. So even when food has not been eaten in a while, stored glucose is released by the liver to maintain adequate blood glucose levels at all times.

When the Process Breaks Down: What Happens with Type 2 Diabetes

When a person has type 2 diabetes, the metabolic process described above does not go according to plan. Exactly why this happens is still not understood, but the result is clear—instead of entering the cells, glucose remains in the bloodstream and blood glucose levels remain high. Why? Because there's either not enough insulin in the bloodstream or the insulin that is there isn't being used well by the body.

Type 2 diabetes doesn't happen all at once. It is a gradual process that generally worsens over time. In a very basic sense, the endocrine system's (the system of organs in the body responsible for making hormones like insulin) insulin-producing ability slowly breaks down.

Why Do I Have Type 2 Diabetes?

Age is a large reason. After time, your body simply doesn't function as well as it once did. But there are other factors involved. Genetics plays a big part. If your parents or grandparents had diabetes, there's a greater chance you'll have diabetes. Race is also a factor. Certain ethnic populations, such as African Americans and Native Americans, run a much higher risk of developing type 2 diabetes. However, two of the biggest contributors to the development of type 2 diabetes are obesity and not getting enough exercise.

Insulin Resistance and Beyond

Not all cases of type 2 diabetes are the same, but for most people, the disease progresses in a similar fashion. There are usually two problems that lead to type 2 diabetes: insulin resistance and insulin deficiency. The first stage is usually insulin resistance. This means the body doesn't respond to insulin properly. There is plenty of insulin in the bloodstream, but the body doesn't use it effectively enough to move the proper amount of glucose into cells. The result is high blood glucose. What follows is a sort of vicious cycle.

During the early phases of insulin resistance, the pancreas can still pump out insulin. The problem is that the body isn't using that insulin correctly and glucose levels stay high. Because glucose levels are high, the body thinks it needs to make more insulin, so it does. Now the body is making much more insulin than it normally would to keep blood glucose levels down. This continues until the pancreas finally can't keep up with the demand. Essentially, the pancreas's ability to make insulin burns out. As type 2 diabetes progresses, insulin production drops, the insulin that is there isn't being used properly, and glucose levels in the blood soar even higher. To make matters worse, in the absence of adequate insulin, the liver continues to release glucose into the bloodstream. This extra glucose adds to the already high levels in the blood.

Eventually, glucose levels will rise to continually abnormal levels. Once the fasting level of glucose in the blood (the level of glucose when no food has been eaten) reaches 126 mg/dl, a person is officially diagnosed with type 2 diabetes.

Pre-Diabetes

As the name suggests, pre-diabetes is a condition that usually comes before full-blown diabetes. In this condition, blood glucose levels are higher than normal, but not high enough to be considered diabetes. Why is this important? First, some studies have shown that even mild hyperglycemia can cause damage over the long run and lead to an increased risk of heart attack and stroke. Second, being diagnosed with pre-diabetes means there's a very good chance a person could develop type 2 diabetes. Since you or a family member probably has diabetes, it's a good idea to ask your doctor about pre-diabetes for other members of your family. The sooner you or family members make changes to your lifestyles, the better the chances for avoiding diabetes altogether.

This is a very simple and basic description of diabetes. The disease is actually very complex and could never be summed up in a few pages. However, this should give you a basic understanding of how type 2 diabetes develops in your body. Using this basic knowledge of how diabetes works will make it easier to understand how treatments work, what you need to do to manage your disease, and hopefully make motivating yourself to change your lifestyle that much simpler.

Other Forms of Diabetes

Type 2 diabetes is by far the most common form of diabetes. Nearly 95% of the people with diabetes have type 2. However, many people, even those with diabetes, can get confused about what type of diabetes they have and how it differs from other forms of the disease. To help clear the air, I'll briefly discuss the other forms of diabetes and how they affect the body.

Type 1 Diabetes

Type 1 diabetes is sometimes called "juvenile diabetes," because nearly all people are diagnosed with the disease in childhood. Even though the consequences of type 1—high blood glucose levels—are the same as those for type 2, the conditions are actually very different.

In common cases of type 1 diabetes, the body's autoimmune system attacks and destroys the beta cells in the pancreas, the cells that produce insulin. Suddenly, the body can no longer make its own insulin and blood glucose levels skyrocket. To survive, people with type 1 diabetes must take injections of insulin.

Gestational Diabetes

Gestational diabetes is a form of diabetes that only affects women who are pregnant and then disappears a few weeks or months after the baby is born. Pregnancy can drastically change the hormones in a woman's body and this can sometimes lead to high blood glucose levels. Women who have gestational diabetes must take steps to control their blood glucose levels to avoid an increased risk for birth defects and other complications. Women who have gestational diabetes also run a much greater risk of developing type 2 diabetes later in life.

COMPLICATIONS OF DIABETES

One of the main hurdles I've encountered with patients in my clinic is the feeling that high blood glucose levels just aren't very dangerous. More than a few times I've heard a patient say he or she just has a "touch of the sugar." I try my best to change this attitude, but it's easy to understand how it develops. At first, diabetes doesn't have many symptoms. Other than situations like extreme hyperglycemia (such as the woman in the beginning of this chapter), there really isn't much pain or discomfort in having elevated blood sugars, so it's natural to assume that nothing is wrong. Over the years, however, high blood glucose levels can cause a variety of very serious health problems, or complications. These complications are what make diabetes a very serious disease. They're also the reason why good blood glucose control is essential.

Heart Disease and Stroke

Scientific studies show that having diabetes is like already having one heart attack. The risk for heart disease, also known as cardiovascular disease, and stroke are that great. In fact, cardiovascular disease kills more people with diabetes than all of the other complications combined.

Many of the risk factors for heart disease are the same as the risk factors for diabetes—mainly obesity, inactivity, and age. To make matters worse, high levels of blood glucose actually damage cells in the blood vessels. Over time, this damage to the cells can lead to arteriosclerosis, or hardening of the arteries. This condition is one of the biggest contributors to heart attack and stroke.

Steps for Prevention

Fortunately, there are a variety of steps you can take to prevent or lessen your risk for heart disease and stroke.

- Control your blood glucose. Keeping your blood glucose in the target range (see the next section, "Diabetes Goals," for specific numbers) is the best way to prevent damage to the cells in your circulatory system.
- If you smoke, quit.
- If you're not getting regular exercise, try to work in at least three 30-minute sessions of activity a week, with the goal of building up to five sessions a week.
- Follow the meal planning recommendations in this book and cut down on foods that are high in fat, especially saturated fat.
- Control your blood pressure and cholesterol.

Just taking these modest steps can go a long way toward preventing some of the deadliest complications of the cardiovascular system.

Neuropathy

Neuropathy is damage to the nerve cells in your body caused by high blood glucose levels over a long period of time. While it can take years for the symptoms of neuropathy to appear, by the time symptoms arrive, much of the damage has already been done.

Neuropathy affects the peripheral nerves, which are the nerves not in the brain or the spinal cord. There are three types of peripheral nerves:

- Motor—these nerves control your voluntary movements, like standing up or moving your arm. Neuropathy can damage these nerves and make it harder to move.
- Sensory—these nerves help you touch and feel senses such as heat, cold, pain, or texture. Damage to these nerves can cause numbness, pain, and loss of feeling.
- Autonomic—the nerves that control involuntary activities, such as breathing, digesting, and regulating heart beat. Damage to autonomic nerves makes it hard for your body's organs to operate properly.

Neuropathy can damage all three types of peripheral nerves.

The symptoms of neuropathy are different depending on the types of nerves being damaged. Motor and sensory nerve damage is usually found in the feet, legs, and sometimes the hands and produces symptoms such as numbness, pain, burning, tingling, weakness, and overly sensitive skin. Damage to the autonomic nerves affects how your organs operate and produces more subtle symptoms, such as diarrhea, constipation, pounding heart rate, dizziness, bladder control problems, and impotence. If you ever have any of these symptoms, talk to your doctor and have a check for nerve damage.

Ulcers and Amputation

You may have heard horror stories about diabetes causing foot and leg amputations. Unfortunately, ulcers and amputations are some of the most difficult consequences of living with neuropathy and vascular disease for years. But they don't have to be. With good blood sugar control and proper attention to your feet and legs, amputations can be avoided.

Foot ulcers start as open wounds on the foot that go untreated. These wounds can be caused by a variety of things, such as wearing shoes that don't fit or walking around barefoot. Normally, ulcers are very painful, so they get noticed, but for those with neuropathy, loss of feeling in the feet numbs this pain. In addition, those with diabetes often also have diminished blood flow to their legs and a greater difficulty in fighting infections, which also contributes to the development and progression of ulcers. If wounds in a person with diabetes are left untreated, they can become infected, which can lead to permanent tissue death and gangrene. Once this occurs, the only treatment may be amputation.

Steps for Prevention

- Control your blood glucose. This is the absolute best thing you can do to prevent neuropathy. In fact, getting your blood glucose levels down and keeping them down can slightly reverse some of the damage to your nerves.
- Quit smoking. Almost all people with diabetes who need amputations are smokers.
- Drink less alcohol. Drinking too much alcohol can cause nerve damage on its own. If you already suffer from neuropathy, it can make it worse.
- Take care of your feet. Wear socks and shoes that fit and do a daily foot check for sores, cuts, and blisters. Do not cut off corns and calluses on your own.
- Control your blood pressure and cholesterol. Preventing damage to and blockage of your blood vessels helps ensure adequate blood flow to your feet.

Kidney Disease

Kidney disease is also known as nephropathy (not to be confused with neuropathy). While it is usually more serious in people with type 1 diabetes, it can also develop in those with type 2, especially if you've had the disease for many years.

Simply put, your kidneys clean your blood. Blood flows through filters in your kidneys, which clean out wastes while leaving in the good and useful things your body needs. High levels of glucose in the blood cause this system to break down. At first, the kidneys become overworked by the extra glucose in the blood. After a while, some of the filters begin to leak a protein called albumin—something your kidneys are supposed to retain—into the urine. As the disease progresses, more and more albumin leaks into the urine and symptoms such as bloating, swelling, and shortness of breath may start to appear. Eventually, some of these leaky filters finally just give out, causing the remaining good filters to shoulder the extra load. Finally, even the good filters begin to fail and wastes in the blood rise to toxic levels. This failure of the kidneys is known as end-stage renal disease, and at this point, you need either a kidney transplant or dialysis to survive.

As with the other complications of diabetes, once the symptoms of kidney disease appear, the disease has already progressed to a pretty bad stage. The key is preventing kidney failure before it's too late.

Steps for Prevention

- Control your blood glucose. I'm starting to sound like a broken record, aren't I? But good blood glucose control can help prevent blood vessel damage, overworking the kidneys, and other conditions that may cause or speed up the development of kidney disease.
- Have your doctor check your kidneys. There are a variety of tests that can detect kidney disease. Treating kidney disease before symptoms show up is the best way to keep it from getting worse.
- Control your blood pressure. High blood pressure causes your kidneys to work harder, which can make damage even worse.

Retinopathy

Retinopathy is one of three eye diseases that routinely affect people with diabetes, the other two being glaucoma and cataracts. Of the three, retinopathy is the most common.

Retinopathy is basically damage to blood vessels in the retina, which is the lining in the back of the eye that senses light. These small blood vessels bring oxygen to the eye, and the damage caused by high levels of glucose can produce some bad results. In mild cases, vessels will bulge and weaken, leaking a little fluid into the eye but not causing any real symptoms. If a lot of fluid leaks into the eye, the eye can swell. If the swelling happens around the center of the eye, the result can be blurred or distorted vision. If damage to vessels in the eye is severe, new vessels will begin growing. These new vessels will spread across the eye and are generally very weak. They can break and hemorrhage in the eye, causing blurred vision and floating spots. They may also spur the growth of scar tissue, which can pull the retina from the back of the eye. This detached retina will cause you to see a large dark area or shadow and, if not treated, will lead to blindness.

Once again, treating retinopathy before symptoms appear is the best way to avoid losing your vision. If have any of the following symptoms, see your doctor immediately:

- Blurry vision
- Floating spots
- Trouble reading
- Shadows or dark areas in your vision
- Trouble seeing at night
- Straight lines appearing curved

Steps for Prevention

- You guessed it—control your blood glucose levels. High blood glucose levels can't damage your eyes if you're keeping your glucose in the target ranges.
- Quit smoking.
- Control your blood pressure and cholesterol. High blood pressure and high cholesterol can make eye disease worse.
- Have a yearly dilated eye exam. Damage to the blood vessels in your eye can happen without any symptoms. The earlier damage is detected, the better the chance that you can save your sight.

Facing the Truth

Talking about the complications of diabetes is not pleasant, and honestly, it can be a little frightening. You've been presented with a long list of nasty conditions, and these are just the most common complications of diabetes. But, like I said before, I'm not trying to scare you. Scare tactics don't work or motivate people to change their lifestyle; instead, they tend to make people just ignore the issues altogether. It's easier to pretend something bad simply isn't there. I don't want that to happen. The task I've set for myself with this book is simple—don't use gimmicks, just be honest, and be straightforward.

That said, complications are part of the reality of diabetes and they need to be understood. Simply put, they are the reason you need to lose weight and control your blood glucose levels. Hopefully, by giving just a brief glimpse into how high levels of blood glucose affect your body, I've helped you make the idea of complications more understandable and more real.

DIABETES GOALS

Now it's time to discuss what goals you should be working toward in terms of your diabetes care. I mentioned earlier that diabetes and numbers go hand in hand, and that's true. There are a lot of numbers you need to remember. Here are some of the most important.

Blood Glucose Goals

Basically, you should aim to keep your blood glucose levels as close to normal (in other words, as close to the glucose levels in people without diabetes) as you can. This isn't easy, and it isn't always possible. On an hourly and daily basis, blood glucose numbers can be very erratic. There will be days when your glucose will be right on target, and then the next day, without any changes in your treatment, they'll be very high for seemingly no reason. The key is to think in the long term. Your average glucose levels, as shown by testing your A1C (see below), are what are important.

The following numbers are suggested goals for people with diabetes. The fasting and postprandial (a fancy way of saying "after eating") numbers represent the milligrams of glucose in one deciliter of blood plasma, which is often shortened to mg/dl. Don't worry; you won't need to remember this. Whenever you check your glucose with a blood glucose monitor, the readings will be in plasma mg/dl. A1C is represented by percentage points.

Keep in mind that no two people are alike, and not everyone will have the same goals. To determine exactly what your blood glucose goals should be, talk with your doctor.

Fasting Plasma Glucose

Fasting plasma glucose is the level of glucose in your blood when you have gone eight hours without eating. For people with diabetes, this should be **between 90 and 130 mg/dl**.

Postprandial Plasma Glucose

Postprandial glucose is the level of glucose in your blood after you have eaten a meal. Because you've just eaten food, this will be higher. Aim for **less than 180 mg/dl**.

A1C

A1C is short for hemoglobin A1c. This number is a little different from your other blood glucose numbers. Instead of telling you what your glucose is at that moment, an A1C reading is more like a gauge of what your glucose readings have been over the past three months. An A1C test is the best way to determine how well your diabetes treatment therapy has been working on average. Your doctor will conduct most A1C checks, but new home-checking kits have just been made available.

In people who don't have diabetes, A1C levels range from 4 to 6%. These are very difficult levels for some people with diabetes to reach. Briefly, the higher a person's A1C level, the higher average blood sugar they have. Therefore, people with diabetes should strive for the lowest possible A1C level they can achieve. The recommended A1C goal for people with diabetes is **less than 7%**.

Blood Pressure Goals

It would be an overstatement to say that controlling your blood pressure is as important as controlling your blood glucose. But it's

Diabetes Goals

A1C	<7%
Fasting Glucose	90–130 mg/dl
After-Meal Glucose	<180 mg/dl
Blood Pressure	<130/80 mmHg
LDL Cholesterol	<100 mg/dl
HDL Cholesterol	>40 mg/dl
Triglycerides	<150 mg/dl

close. High blood pressure, also known as hypertension, worsens an already high risk for heart attack and aggravates nearly every complication of diabetes, from neuropathy to retinopathy. If you have diabetes, you simply must control your blood pressure.

Because high blood pressure poses such a dangerous risk for people with diabetes, blood pressure goals are a little more stringent than they are for the rest of the population. If you have diabetes, strive to keep your blood pressure **less than 130/80 mmHg**.

There are a variety of effective blood pressure medications available, but I always tell my patients that changing your diet and starting an exercise regimen are the cheapest and easiest ways to get blood pressure under control. Talk to your doctor about the best methods for you.

Cholesterol and Other Blood Lipid Goals

The fats in your blood are called lipids, and the same rules that apply to blood pressure apply to lipids: if you have diabetes, you need to control your levels of cholesterol and blood fats in order to avoid or lessen the progression of complications.

Not all blood fats are the same. There are three to which you must pay close attention—LDL cholesterol, HDL cholesterol, and triglycerides. LDL cholesterol is an abbreviation for "low-density lipoprotein" and is often referred to as "bad" cholesterol. You want to keep your LDL cholesterol as low as possible. HDL cholesterol is "high-density lipoprotein" and is often called "good" cholesterol. The more HDL cholesterol in your blood, the better. Triglycerides are another form of blood fat you need to watch. Like LDL cholesterol, you want to keep your level of triglycerides as low as possible.

So what lipid levels should you shoot for? Following are the ADA's recommendations:

LDL Cholesterol	Less than 100 mg/dl
HDL Cholesterol	More than 40 mg/dl, perhaps higher for women
Triglycerides	Less than 150 mg/dl

Like blood pressure, there are a variety of medications available to treat high cholesterol and other blood fats. And once again, changing your diet to foods low in cholesterol and saturated fat and starting an exercise regimen are two of the easiest, most readily available treatments for high lipids.

TREATMENTS FOR TYPE 2 DIABETES

So far in this chapter we've discussed, in a simplified form, how diabetes affects your body. We've explored the different complications that can develop if diabetes and blood glucose levels are not controlled. We've talked about the numbers and goals that you as a person with diabetes should strive toward. What we haven't discussed, though, is how you actually manage your blood glucose. I've saved a brief discussion of this for last.

There's no one way to manage diabetes. There are many treatments available and many combinations of treatments as well. Choosing the right combination of management methods for you is the key to good glucose control. There is no single path, no magic bullet, no true cure. But there are a variety of things you can do to control your blood glucose levels well enough that it's almost like not having diabetes at all. It's not always going to be easy and there will be ups and downs. But diabetes is one of the few chronic conditions you can control. It's all a matter of commitment to being and staying healthy.

Oral Medications

Most people diagnosed with type 2 diabetes are prescribed oral medications if diet and exercise aren't enough to control blood glucose levels. Keep in mind that oral medications are meant to complement diet and exercise, not replace them. Just popping a few pills may not get your blood glucose levels under control.

Right now there are five types of oral diabetes medications available in the United States, though as pharmaceutical research progresses, there are bound to be more. These five types are:

- **Sulfonylureas**—these help your body send out more of its own insulin, may help your body respond to insulin, and may slow your liver's release of stored insulin into the bloodstream.

- **Biguanides**—these pills cause your liver to release stored glucose more slowly and may also help your body respond to insulin.

- **Alpha-glucosidase inhibitors**—these pills slow the amount of time it takes for your intestines to break down carbohydrate into glucose, causing the glucose to enter your bloodstream more slowly and lessening high glucose levels after meals.

- **Thiazolidinediones**—these drugs make your muscles and fat cells more sensitive to insulin and may reduce the release of glucose stored in your liver.

- **Meglitinides**—like sulfonylureas, these pills help your body send out more insulin, only more quickly and for a short time.

All oral diabetes medications carry the risk of side effects. The side effects for each drug are different and should be considered before you start any oral medication treatment. Talk with your doctor for more information.

Insulin

The insulin used to treat diabetes is not the same as the insulin your pancreas produces. In other words, you're not injecting human insulin into your bloodstream. However, the insulin used by people with diabetes is a synthetic form of the hormone, and it produces the same results—it helps move glucose into your cells.

After being diagnosed with type 2 diabetes, many of my patients ask me, sometimes in a panic, if they'll have to start taking daily shots of insulin. I reassure them that this usually isn't necessary in the early stages of the disease. Type 2 diabetes is not like type 1, where you need to take several insulin shots a day just to survive. Most newly diagnosed patients begin with diet and exercise, and perhaps oral medications. However, that doesn't mean you will never need to take injections of insulin.

Sometimes, diet, exercise, and oral medications just aren't enough. If these treatments don't get blood glucose levels under control, insulin may be necessary. Also, and this is one of the cold, hard facts of diabetes, the disease will get harder to manage over time. After many years with diabetes, your pancreas simply will not produce enough insulin, and oral medications won't be able to get glucose levels into the target ranges. At this time, insulin will be necessary. Some of my patients are disheartened by this, until I remind them that this can be a great motivator to start taking care of themselves and fend off the need for insulin until much later down the road.

What Goes Up Can Come Down: Hypoglycemia

We have discussed how having high blood glucose levels—hyperglycemia—over long periods of time can lead to the complications that make diabetes so dangerous. In the short term, isolated low blood glucose, called hypoglycemia, can also be dangerous. Hypoglycemia occurs when your blood glucose is less than 70 mg/dl or drops low enough to cause symptoms that are not normal during a typical day. Because diabetes medications, particularly sulfonylureas, meglitinides, and insulin, are so powerful at lowering blood sugar, sometimes the dose that someone takes at a particular time causes their blood glucose to drop too low. Here are some important points regarding hypoglycemia.

1. Taking diabetes medication, particularly short-acting insulin, without eating can lead to hypoglycemia. Diabetes medications, especially insulin, work best when used with a predictable, stable meal plan. Make sure that you discuss the proper timing of your medication with your doctor or health care team.

2. The symptoms of hypoglycemia can be subtle and vary from person to person, but often include sweating, nausea, lightheadedness, fatigue, and headache. More severe symptoms include blurred vision, confusion, passing out, seizures, and even death. Over time, many people lose the ability to recognize the symptoms of hypoglycemia. We call this *hypoglycemia unawareness*, and it can be a very dangerous condition.

3. When in doubt about hypoglycemia—go ahead and treat it (see below for more on how to treat hypoglycemia). Because of the dangerous nature of hypoglycemia, if you simply feel like you might be low, go ahead and have a snack. Ideally, you'll want to test your blood glucose, and then treat hypoglycemia with the 15-15 rule (see page 34).

4. A person with diabetes should also encourage his or her friends and loved ones to have training in treating hypoglycemic reactions because a person who is hypoglycemic may become confused and not be able to treat him- or herself.

5. Certain people, particularly those on insulin, carry a syringe with them containing glucagon—the hormone that counteracts insulin. If such a person falls into an unarousable or confused state, family members should know how to mix and inject glucagon immediately.

6. If you are having repeated episodes of hypoglycemia, discuss medication changes with your doctor or health care team. Sometimes

continued on page 34

continued from page 33

as patients make healthy changes in their diet or lose weight, their medication programs become too powerful and need to be adjusted. Having more than a rare, mild hypoglycemic event indicates a need for changes in the medical program.

How to Treat Hypoglycemia: The 15-15 Rule

1. Check your blood glucose with a meter, if you can. If your blood glucose is under 70 mg/dl, go to steps 2 and 3. If you can't check, go to steps 2 and 4.

2. Eat or drink something with about 15 grams (1/2 oz) of carbohydrate. Foods with 15 grams of carbohydrate are listed below.

3. Wait 15–20 minutes, and then check again.

   If your blood glucose is still under 70 mg/dl after this period, repeat steps 2 and 3. If you have repeated steps 2 and 3 and your blood glucose is still under 70 mg/dl, call your doctor or have someone take you to a hospital emergency room. You may need outside help in treating your low blood glucose or something else may be causing these signs.

   If your blood glucose has risen over 70 mg/dl, stop drinking and/or eating the foods listed for treating hypoglycemia. You may still feel the symptoms of hypoglycemia even after your blood glucose has gone back up. Go to step 4.

4. If your next meal is more than an hour away, eat a small snack of carbohydrate and protein. Try a slice of bread with reduced-fat peanut butter or six crackers with low-fat cheese.

Foods Used to Treat Hypoglycemia

- 3–4 glucose tablets or a 15-gram carbohydrate tube of glucose gel (the dosage is printed on the package)
- 1/2 cup (4 oz) fruit juice
- 1/3 can (4 oz) regular (not sugar-free) soda
- 1 cup (8 oz) nonfat milk
- 2 tablespoons of raisins (40 to 50)
- 3 graham cracker squares
- 1 tablespoon granulated sugar
- 6 saltine crackers
- 1 tablespoon honey or syrup

The Cheapest, Safest, Most Accessible Form of Treatment: Diet and Exercise

This is my favorite therapy for controlling type 2 diabetes. You don't need health insurance to get it, it's readily available, it has an immediate positive impact on your blood glucose levels, and it's safe for everyone. It's healthy eating and exercise.

Many people don't realize the impact losing weight through diet and exercise has on their overall health. If you have high blood pressure, losing weight will help. If you run a high risk for cardio-vascular disease (and if you have diabetes, you do), losing weight will help. If you're having trouble meeting your blood glucose goals, losing weight will definitely help. Just losing as little as 10 pounds is enough to improve your diabetes control. The first pre-scription I write for a newly diagnosed diabetes patient in my clin-ic? Lose weight.

But let's be honest. I doubt any of this is news to you. You prob-ably know that losing weight is good for you. That's why the title of this section doesn't say the "Easiest Form of Treatment." We've all tried to drop a few pounds and guess what? It's really hard to do. Even if we have success in the beginning, over time we fall back into our old habits, the extra weight creeps back on, and we're back to where we started, if not worse. And the older you get, the hard-er it gets. Old habits die hard.

Why does this happen? There are a lot of reasons, and I try to cover as many as I can in the rest of this book. A lot of it has to do with bad habits we pick up early and carry with us the rest of our lives. An even bigger factor is that we approach dieting in the wrong way and set ourselves up for failure. We focus on the short term, follow eating plans that are so restrictive we could never fol-low them for more than a few months, and then after some initial success, slip right back into our old ways of eating and exercising. And this isn't completely our fault—this is how we've been taught to diet by an industry that thrives on short-term success and long-term failure. Finally, we're surrounded by temptation, from outside and within.

The goal of this book is to help you begin your diabetes weight-loss therapy treatment and follow it for the rest of your life. There won't be any gimmicks, but there will be a lot of self-evaluation and a lot of cold, hard truth. Hopefully, by following the advice in here, the same advice I've seen work with the patients in my clinic time and time again, you'll end up with a healthier you. You'll look better, you'll feel better, you'll have better control of your blood glucose, and your risk for several complications will be lower. The rest of this book is devoted to starting you on this effective course of treatment.

SECTION HIGHLIGHTS
A Brief Summary of Important Points
Discussed in this Section

1. Obesity levels in the United States have grown to almost epidemic proportions. Because obesity and overweight are risk factors for diabetes, the number of people diagnosed with type 2 diabetes has risen as well.

2. Diabetes is a complex disorder that affects how the body obtains and uses energy from a sugar called glucose. Glucose is in many of the foods we eat, but a lot of it comes from carbohydrate-heavy foods.

3. Complications are conditions that develop after years of elevated blood glucose. There are lots of complications of diabetes, and many are life threatening. Most of what people associate with diabetes are in fact the complications of diabetes, such as amputations, heart attacks, etc.

4. Being overweight or obese makes controlling blood glucose harder, which puts you at a higher risk of developing dangerous complications. These risks can be reduced by losing weight and keeping healthy.

5. Because it is hard to see or feel the effects diabetes has on our bodies, there is no immediate incentive to take care of ourselves. This is one of the most dangerous aspects of the disease.

6. To stay healthy, you need to strive toward diabetes goals and pay attention to your diabetes care numbers, such as blood glucose levels, blood pressure readings, and cholesterol levels.

7. Losing weight through diet and exercise is one of the best ways to improve your blood glucose.

Step One:

Thinking About Your Eating Habits

Chapter 4
How Do You Eat?

How do you eat? This may sound like a strange question, but this is one of the keys to losing weight over the long term. Too many diets, especially fad diets, only focus on *what* you eat or changing your eating patterns for a short period of time and not on *how* you normally eat. Plenty of people think dieting means not eating anything for a few weeks (or packing yourself so full of meat that you can't eat anything else) and then returning to the "old ways." We've all tried it, and exactly how successful was this? The typical "lose weight fast" diets aren't going to work in the long term or keep your diabetes numbers in the healthy range. Therefore, the first thing you need to do is actually figure out how you eat.

In thinking about how you eat, we're not going to focus specifically on what or how much you eat (though this is a part of it); instead, I'm asking you to think about your *eating habits*. Eating habits are those little things we do while we are eating or just before we eat. Habits are those things we do for so long that we no longer even notice we're doing them. We also have habits that surround how we eat, and they can often be hidden contributors to weight gain and failed diet attempts.

Eating Habits

Here is a short list of questions about some common eating habits. There are many more, and everyone has different habits. Use these as a foundation for examining your own eating behaviors.

- Do you always have a snack while watching TV?
- Does all food need sauce or gravy?
- Is a second or third serving for a meal automatic?
- Do many of your social activities revolve around eating?
- Do you tend to order the bigger meal because it is a better deal?
- Do you eat when you are nervous?
- Do you eat because you are bored?
- Do you eat before bed?
- Do you eat your food faster than other people around you?
- Do you usually eat food out of containers rather than putting it on a plate?
- Do you ever feel out of control when eating?
- Do you skip breakfast and overeat later in the day?

More than likely you answered yes to a couple of these. This is not surprising. Most Americans would answer "yes" to many of these questions, and just as many would admit they didn't know these behaviors were connected to their weight gain. Recognizing these bad habits is the first step to making long-term change.

SELF-EVALUATION

Thinking about eating habits and how you eat is the first step in the 1-2-3 Diabetes Diet, and it's a hard one. It requires self-evaluation. You're going to have to look at yourself and at behaviors you have never even considered and identify parts of your lifestyle that you can change.

Self-Evaluation? For a Diet?

Many companies ask their employees to do self-evaluations of their performances, asking workers to point out all of their successes and identify areas of improvement. Your job may do this, too, so this process may be familiar. The 1-2-3 Diabetes Diet asks you to do the very same thing. However, "self-evaluation" sounds a little clinical. Another word you can use to describe this step is *soul-searching*. Neither activity is easy, but I think everyone gains from such a tough task. It requires willpower, objectivity, and dedication.

Food Diary

You can do some little things to make this task easier. You should jot down your daily eating habits on a notepad, describing what you eat, when you eat it, and what you are doing at the time. This is often called a food diary, and I ask all of my patients who need to lose weight to use one. I've even included one at the end of this chapter. You can use that one or make your own. A food diary doesn't have to be anything special. You can buy a memo pad from your local pharmacy or grocery store. Blank sheets of paper stapled together will work just as well, as long as you can keep it relatively organized. Regardless, writing down what you do so you have a record of it will be very helpful. Sometimes we forget the simplest things.

Other tactics include talking to friends and family about your eating habits or even having them watch your behavior and write it down. The only problem with doing this is that if these people have the same habits, they may not notice them in you. Another thing you can do is to put your food diary on a computer; that way you can type up the information every night. For those of you feeling particularly modern, there are food diary programs available for home computers and handheld computers. However, using a computer has its pros and cons. You'll probably still have to jot down information on slips of paper (don't rely on your memory to do all of the work for you), but in typing the information on a computer, you get to see the facts again and can look at them with more objectivity. Reviewing your entries by re-reading them or typing them out later will let you think more clearly about your eating habits.

The most important thing to keep in mind at this point is that you're taking a step in the right direction. You may have moments when you don't want to add entries to your food diary. You may also become discouraged by what you discover. Don't let this get you down. Sometimes doing the best thing for your health and future involves a few missteps. Have you ever tried to quit smoking? That's a really difficult task, and it often takes several tries to get on a successful pace.

There is one cardinal sin when it comes to food diaries—jotting down false entries. You may think at the moment that you're simply getting your doctor or health care team or your spouse off your back, but in reality, you're just hurting yourself. You're lying to yourself, too, which is the worst part of that idea. Be patient. Keep an open mind. Accept that this is a difficult task and that the big thing right now is that you're starting to make changes for a better, healthier future.

Keeping healthy, especially when you have diabetes, can be a difficult task, so you should be proud that you've even gone this far. Don't give up. Remember that you're doing this for yourself and your family, not your doctor, not your health care team, and certainly not for me.

Food Diary 101

This will probably be a surprising activity because very few of us are truly aware of how much our eating habits affect how much, what, and when we eat. Keeping a food diary will motivate you and prepare you for change and, ultimately, success in weight loss.

At first, a food diary may seem to take too much time. You will soon realize how helpful it is to know exactly the amount and types of foods you are eating and what you are doing while you eat. Change can begin once you decide to become more aware of your eating patterns. After you make changes in your eating patterns, you will use the food diary less or not at all. Remember, you're keeping this food diary:

- To identify the situations and circumstances of how you eat
- To determine how many calories or servings you are eating
- To help you find the easiest way to begin cutting back on your calorie intake
- To help you become an expert at counting calories and following a meal plan

We'll get into calorie counting later on. In the meantime, eat as you normally do (which can be very hard when you're keeping a diary, since your natural inclination is to eat better than usual. Remember, be honest with yourself!) and record this information in your food diary until you feel you have enough details to become aware of your eating patterns. This should usually take at least a week to get a good idea of your habits. But even when you begin using meal plans, you should keep up on your food diary to see where you can make improvements in the future and where you are currently making improvements. After an extended period, you'll find that you need your food diary less and less and can gradually stop using it if you feel that it is no longer useful.

What to Record in Your Food Diary

In your food diary, make columns or rows for the following information:

- Date
- Time you eat
- Meal or snack you had
- Servings or how much you eat
- Your mood when you eat
- How hungry you felt before you ate

- Number of calories or servings of each food
- Other activities you were doing while you were eating, such as watching TV, standing in the kitchen, or driving to work

Look at my sample food diary on pages 44–45 for an idea of how to organize this information. Much of this is pretty straightforward, but some requires a little more thought. Under the heading "Meal/Snack," write down what foods you eat, not just "lunch" or "dinner" or "snack." You're going to need to be very specific. Under the heading "Calories," write down the estimated calories for what you ate (more on this in Chapter 11). Under the heading "Number of Servings," record the number of servings you ate. Use the "Total" boxes at the bottom of your food diary to record the number of calories or food servings for all of the meals in that day. The food diary I've provided is two pages long, and you'll be using both pages for all of your eating in one day.

Three Food Diary Guidelines
1. *Measure how much you eat whenever possible.* Use measuring cups and spoons or calculate the number of servings from the package so that you have an accurate record of what you are eating. Eyeballing a serving size does not work until you have measured the correct sizes for several weeks and are used to seeing and eating them. Of course, you'll be doing a lot of this when cooking and eating at home. When you're eating out, put down an educated guess. There is more about serving sizes in chapter 6.

2. *Write down everything you eat immediately after you eat it.* You need to carry your food diary with you throughout the day to keep track of everything you eat or drink, and I mean *everything*. It doesn't matter if you have a handful of M&Ms, a few crackers, a small glass of juice, or your morning coffee (does it have cream and sugar?); write it all down.

3. *Stay positive.* I think most people have the capacity to make weight loss a tangible goal. A big step in this process is simply thinking about what you're eating and making small changes, which is what a food diary will help you do. By writing down what you eat, it makes you think about your diet. Down the road, making a simple choice between one bag of potato chips and another because you checked the calorie content is a sign that you're thinking about what you're eating. Maybe someday, you'll be so aware that you even pass on the chips and choose some fruits or vegetables. But we all have to start somewhere.

Food Diary (Page 1)

Date: _____

WHAT I ATE

What Food Did I Eat?	Number of Servings	Calories

Total: _____ _____

Food Diary (Page 2)

Date: _____

EATING HABITS

Food and Beverage	Time	What Was I Doing (Who, Where, Situation)	R = Regular Meal B = Binge Meal U = Unplanned Meal	Feelings Before Eating	Hunger (score 1-10, with 1 being not hungry & 10 being starving

Chapter 5
What Do You Eat?

Not only does the 1-2-3 Diabetes Diet require that you think about how you eat, but, as you've probably been expecting, you'll also have to think about what you eat. Just about all of us know, whether we actually acknowledge it or not, that the food we put into our bodies can have a good or bad effect on our overall health. I'm now asking you to spend a little more time thinking about what you eat and taking action to change your eating habits. Hand in hand with this knowledge comes the idea that we should control how much we eat, but we'll talk more about that later.

BASIC NUTRITION

Before we really get started, we should review the basics of nutrition. No matter what meal plan you decide to use, you will need to eat a healthy variety of nutrients to stay fit and healthy.

Calories

You've heard of calories before. Simply enough, calories are a measurement of the amount of energy provided by a food. Calories aren't so different from watts, which we count to determine energy bills. Many different nutrients, including protein, carbohydrate, and fat, provide calories.

Everyone should pay attention to the number of calories they eat because it directly represents how much exercise they need to keep from gaining weight. The more calories you eat, the more you need to burn in order to keep fit and stay at a healthy weight. The less you eat, the less you need to burn. As you can imagine, eating less and burning more is the quickest way to weight loss.

Carbohydrates

The word *carbohydrate* describes many types of nutrients, including starches, sugars, and fiber. You find carbohydrate in many foods, and it plays a key role in your weight and diabetes. All carbohydrates used by the body are eventually broken down into one common substance: glucose. We often refer to glucose as "sugar." As I showed in Chapter 3, glucose is the main fuel the body uses.

Before we go any farther, let's clear up some common misunderstandings about the word "sugar" and its relationship with carbohydrate. Carbohydrates enter our bodies in two forms: sugars and starches. Sugars include glucose, fructose (found in fruit), and lactose (found in milk). Starches enter our body when we eat grains, pasta, and potatoes. Once the body breaks down carbohydrate into glucose, it doesn't care where it came from. It could come from pasta, candy, or a soda—it doesn't matter. This is why the common myth that people with diabetes can't eat "sugar" is not true. A potato can raise blood sugar just as much as a piece of cake. What does matter, however, is *how much* glucose is entering your bloodstream from the meal you just ate. So, when you hear the word "sugar" tossed about, realize that in terms of diabetes, "sugar" is a scientific word that refers to more than just table sugar (sucrose). Calorie for calorie, table sugar raises blood glucose about the same amount as other carbohydrates.

Because carbohydrates are so complex, have such an enormous effect on your blood glucose levels, and are commonly distorted in a number of recent fad diets, I talk about carbohydrates more in depth in Chapter 19.

A Note About Dietary Fiber

Fiber is a part of plant foods that the body cannot digest. A good amount of fiber in your diet can keep you healthy, and it's pretty easy to increase the amount you eat. The general recommendation is to have 25–30 grams of fiber a day. Just about all of us know that you eat fiber when you want to relieve constipation, but here are two more important reasons why we should all have more fiber in our diets.

- Soluble fiber (found in beans, oats, peas, apples, and more) can help lower cholesterol.
- Fiber can help in weight loss. It takes longer to chew, which means

that your body has time to recognize that you are no longer hungry. Meals that contain a lot of fiber feel larger and keep you full longer, which means you will likely eat less food over the course of a day. And even though fiber-rich foods feel larger in your stomach, they usually contain fewer calories than other foods, so that further reduces the calories you eat.

Fiber can be added to your diet in many simple ways. You can find it in whole-grain foods, fruits, beans, and vegetables. Generally, whole-wheat foods have more fiber than others, so if you have a choice, go with whole-wheat bread and pasta to add more fiber to your diet. You should try to add fiber to your diet with food, not with pills, because high-fiber foods provide so many good nutrients in addition to the fiber.

Protein

Protein is an essential part of a healthy diet, as long as it is eaten in moderation. Proteins repair tissue and help form new body tissues.

Protein is found mostly in meat, poultry, and seafood, as well as in dairy products such as milk and cheese. You can also find protein in beans, peas, and lentils. A healthy diet will include about 4–6 ounces of protein-rich food per day (about 10% of your total daily calories). We try to limit how much protein we put in our diets because most of our protein comes from animal foods, which also contain a great deal of fat.

Fat

Fats are what your body prefers to use to store extra energy. In a very simplified way, all of that extra weight sitting around your waist and stomach is energy you ate but didn't burn being stored as fat. In addition to storing fuel, a small amount of fat is necessary to provide essential fatty acids, carry some fat-soluble vitamins, maintain healthy skin, and help produce some hormones. Three types of fat appear in our diet: monounsaturated, polyunsaturated, and saturated.

Health professionals generally consider monounsaturated and polyunsaturated fats the healthiest fats to have in your diet. A variety of oils (olive, sunflower, sesame, vegetable, and corn oils), cereals, and grains contain these fats. A special kind of unsaturated fat, called omega-3 fatty acid (found in fish, flaxseed oil, and some nuts), can provide multiple health benefits, including reduced risk of cardiovascular disease, improved cholesterol levels, and reduced risk of cancer.

The fats to avoid are saturated fats and *trans*-fats. These fats are made by turning liquid into solids through chemical processes. Saturated fats, mainly found in meat and other animal products, can increase rates of cardiovascular disease and worsen cholesterol levels. *Trans*-fats can increase your levels of bad cholesterol and may actually lower your levels of good cholesterol. Therefore, when you select food for your diet, you should avoid saturated fats and *trans*-fats as much as possible, eating none daily if possible. This should be relatively easy; both types of fat are now marked on nutrition labels on foods. You will have to be more careful in restaurants, though. Handy books, such as the American Diabetes Association's *Guide to Healthy Restaurant Eating,* give you all of the nutritional information for meals at common restaurants.

Vitamins and Minerals

You've heard that you should take your vitamins since you were little, and this tidbit of wisdom still applies. Keep in mind that if you maintain a healthy, balanced diet, you won't need to take vitamin pills. The food in your meals will supply just about all of the vitamins you need. Additionally, research suggests that the best way to get vitamins is through the food you eat because your body uses them more efficiently. In certain cases, vitamin supplements will be necessary. Pregnant women, strict vegetarians, and elderly people may benefit from adding more vitamins to their diets. Vitamins are an important part of overall wellness, but because our bodies require such small amounts of them on a daily basis, a healthy, diverse diet should provide all that you need.

Summing Up

All people, with or without diabetes, need a regular supply of all of these nutrients to stay healthy. Diets that are based on eliminating any one of these nutrients altogether are simply not healthy. On the other hand, eating too much of any one of the nutrients is not a healthy way to eat either.

I KNOW I SAID NO FIGURES, BUT...

So now you know the nutrients that make up a healthy diet. Now it's time to begin thinking about how to construct a healthy diet of your own. I realize I said earlier that I wouldn't bog you down with graphs and charts. And I won't. However, there is one figure that I do think is important and that's the new U.S. Department of Agriculture (USDA) My Pyramid plan, which replaces the old food pyramid we grew up with. Below is the general version of the new Pyramid, but this is only a part of the new approach to tailoring nutrition requirements to each individual. The full plan is available online at *www.mypyramid.gov*. I highly encourage you to check it out.

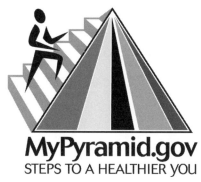

MyPyramid.gov
STEPS TO A HEALTHIER YOU

From left to right, the bars represent the following food groups: grains, vegetables, fruits, oils, milk, and meats and beans. The exact daily serving amounts rely on your age, gender, weight, and activity level, and it is impossible to represent this in a single pyramid (there are 12 total pyramids). To properly use the new USDA food pyramid, visit the website at *http://www.mypyramid.gov*.

I'm showing you the new pyramid here to illustrate how thinking about nutrition has changed over the years. Compared with the old food pyramid, the My Pyramid Plan features a significantly new approach to healthy eating. Most importantly, this new pyramid gives you a personalized food pyramid that is determined by your age, sex, and level of daily physical activity. This is because health professionals have realized over the years that the number of servings a day for each nutrient varies from person to person. Also, notice that no specific food is identified as a "good guy" or "bad guy." Instead, you are given the choice of what foods to include in your diet, which gives you a great amount of freedom and independence in creating your own healthy lifestyle.

Interestingly enough, freedom to create a healthy lifestyle based on your own likes and dislikes just so happens to be a major component of the 1-2-3 Diabetes Diet.

Chapter 6
How Much Do You Eat?

Okay, so I've described why you need to think about how you eat. I've also shown that you need to think about what you eat. Now it's time to think about how much you eat. You don't need to be rocket scientist to figure this out, but how much food you eat has a powerful effect on your overall diet. Moreover, if you have diabetes and want to lose weight and improve your health, you can pretty much forget about eating with abandon. That's right, you can't just eat as much of whatever you want whenever you want when you have diabetes.

PORTION CONTROL

Portion control is a simple commonsense approach to eating. Portion control means that you reduce your serving sizes to the point where you are satisfied but not stuffed. If you control the portions of food that you eat, you are taking a very important step forward in living with a healthy diet.

The best way to guarantee that you continue to eat what you like is to control your portions so that you don't max out on calories, carbohydrate, and everything else by the time you've finished your meal. The huge upside to this is that you will still be able to enjoy most of your favorite foods, just in much smaller portions. Giving up foods we like is usually the biggest sacrifice we make when we take on quick-fix diets. This overwhelming sacrifice almost always leads to failure.

Portion control can be easy; it just requires self-control and some thought about what you put on your plate or order at a restaurant.

You're simply limiting your serving sizes. Keep in mind that this can be more difficult than it appears at first glance. We are constantly treated to very large servings of food in restaurants and many stores offer food in bulk or at least very large quantities. Our bargain-based, bigger-is-better society has shifted our notions of reasonable servings. When was the last time you looked at the serving size on a package of food at a grocery store and laughed out loud because the serving size was incredibly small? Probably not so long ago. This is a lesson in perspective. That seemingly tiny serving is *actually how much you are supposed to eat.* Unfortunately, food comes in such large quantities, whether you're buying it at Costco, Wal-Mart, or Safeway, that sensible portions look and seem ridiculously small. The same happens at restaurants.

Q&A

So what is a "sensible serving" of food?

Usually, when you finish eating a meal, you should not feel hungry anymore but you should not feel stuffed either. You should be able to move easily and feel awake. When you become full, stop eating—no matter how much food is left on your plate. Save the leftovers for another meal. If you're also taking care of diabetes, it is especially important that you have a balanced diet that will keep your blood glucose under control. Therefore, you should mix your meals with healthy serving sizes of many different foods to make sure you get the right amount of nutrients and vitamins from every meal.

The table below should help you figure out how much one serving of each of these foods should be.

One Serving of Food	Equals
Fresh fruit or vegetables	1 cup
Canned fruit or cooked vegetables	1/2 cup
Starchy vegetables or dried beans	1/2 cup
Bread	1 slice
Dry cereal	3/4 cup
Cooked cereal	1/2 cup
Rice or pasta	1/3 cup
Dairy products (e.g., milk or yogurt)	1 cup
Lean meats, chicken, and fish	3 ounces
Oil, margarine, or butter	1 teaspoon

These portions seem small, don't they? Well, they're not. They seem tiny because our ideas of what a portion or a serving should be have grown to unhealthy levels.

A Few Beginning Steps in Portion Control

- You don't need to eat everything on your plate. Food is plentiful these days, perhaps too plentiful.
- Try to cut down on snacks, especially if you're just eating out of boredom or while sitting at the computer or watching TV.
- Start looking at what you are eating and make small but healthier changes. For example, if you have a bagel for breakfast every day, pick up some light cream cheese instead of the full, fatty kind. If you love movie theater popcorn, try it with no butter. These might not seem like much, but small changes add up to hundreds of calories a day that you've cut from your diet without leaving you feeling deprived.

Has Big Gotten Bigger?

The U.S. National Heart, Lung, and Blood Institute has put together a nifty little quiz that shows how much serving sizes have increased over the past 20 years. It shows you a picture of a typical serving from the past and compares it, side by side, with today's typical serving size. The quiz is on the Internet at *http:// hin.nhlbi.nih.gov/portion*. I highly recommend checking it out for a good lesson in perspective.

Seeing Sensible Servings

It's important when you first start to control your portions that you use measuring cups, scales, and other tools that allow you to be as precise as possible. As you progress, though, your ability to "eyeball" servings will improve. Of course, when you're in a restaurant or not serving the food yourself, you have no choice but to estimate how big a serving is. Following are some good guidelines.

- A 1/2-cup serving of canned fruit, vegetables, or potatoes looks like half of a tennis ball sitting on your plate.
- 3 ounces of meat, fish, or chicken is about the size of a deck of playing cards or the palm of your hand.
- A 1-ounce serving of cheese is about the size of your thumb.
- A 1-cup serving of milk, yogurt, or fresh greens is about the size of your fist.
- 1 teaspoon of oil is about the size of your thumb tip.

Restaurant Tips

Constantly eating out at restaurants is the easiest way to sabotage a healthy eating plan. Not only are you in the dark on calorie and nutrient content, but you also have no control over ingredients or servings. Still, eating out is a lot of fun and this diet would be way too rigid if I suggested you cut it out completely. This topic is covered in more detail in Chapter 25. Instead, try these little tricks to cut down on your calories when eating out.

- Eat half of your meal and take the rest home for lunch tomorrow.
- Split an entrée or dessert with a friend.
- Ask for substitutions. For example, ask for steamed vegetables or a salad instead of French fries.
- Ask for all sauces, dressings, and gravy on the side and use only a small amount.

But...It's Just a Cheeseburger

Let's use what we have learned about healthy eating to evaluate a simple example of a typical fast food meal. Not one of those small ones, mind you, but one of those double-decker fried deals you can get with an order of fries and a great big soda.

How you eat: If you're eating this cheeseburger out of habit rather than hunger, you're adding unnecessary calories to your daily intake. Maybe it's lunchtime at work, but you had a big or late breakfast. You're not really hungry, but your friends are going to grab some food and you don't want to be stuck at work when you don't have to be there. Maybe you're hitting the drive-thru on the way home from work because it's late and you're too tired to cook something healthier at home. Regardless, these are eating habits that can be changed.

What you eat: This cheeseburger isn't the healthiest option for a meal—it is too high in nutrients you don't need (saturated fat, cholesterol, sodium) and low in nutrients that the American diet typically doesn't provide (fiber, whole grains, healthy fats). Are there other options at this restaurant that are smaller and even slightly healthier?

How much you eat: You want fries with that burger? Or maybe you're going to have two burgers. You want the giant soda instead of that puny regular-size one? You may feel hungry or you may just be eating this much because it tastes so good. The fact is that your typical fast food "value meal" contains enough calories, protein, carbohydrate, and fat to feed a person for an entire day! Think about what this does to your body, to your blood glucose levels, to your heart. If this trend continues, what will it do to your overall health? Think of all that extra energy your body is storing away as fat. The human body simply was not designed to eat this much in one sitting, day in and day out. Getting a smaller soda, fries, and burger can still fill you up and not be as unhealthy. An even better option would be to order a whole-grain sandwich or wrap (yes, with vegetables) with a small side salad and bottled water (or flavored mineral water).

Chapter 7
The Number One, Most Important Concept in this Book

So far in this section I've presented the three basic questions you need to ask yourself to evaluate your situation and kick start the weight loss process: How do you eat? What do you eat? How much do you eat? By answering these three questions, you will come closer to long-term weight loss than you probably ever have before. Why? Because you have taken one fundamental step that almost every other diet ignores. You are thinking about your eating behavior instead of simply eating different foods and following a set-in-stone plan. This is why almost all diets fail, because they focus on the food and not the person. This is like treating a brain tumor with aspirin because it gives you a headache. Don't treat the symptom, treat the cause. The key to long-term success is changing those things that cause you to make poor food choices, not necessarily the bad food itself. But what are those things? While there are many factors that cause us to make these poor food choices, there is one that stands out—self-control.

SELF-CONTROL

It's time to talk about self-control. As you will see, I believe achieving self-control is the key to achieving good health. Self-control is at times a difficult thing to accomplish. We all like to enjoy ourselves. Ultimately, life is full of urges and desires. Thankfully, in civilized society, people have learned how to balance and control these urges; otherwise, the world would be in utter chaos.

There are many real-life examples of self-control. For example, many people would love to sleep in every day. This is a powerful urge. The reality is that, thankfully, most of us get up and do what is required of us on a daily basis, whether it is going to work or to school. Sexual desire is another powerful urge that most people must understand and control. Many of us desire more money and material possessions, yet thankfully most people don't just steal and rob others to get what they want.

Eating is also a powerful force and can be difficult to control. But just as we have seen that other urges and desires need to be controlled, why should the desire to eat be any different? Sure, it would be fun to gorge at every meal, but we all know deep in our hearts that this would ultimately be unhealthy. As I have said before, I am convinced that most people already know the basics about overall good nutrition and portion control. So why is it that so many people fail to control the urge to overeat?

Fighting Yourself

Why is self-control so hard? There are a lot of reasons, too many to fit within this book. That's like asking, "Why do people do things that are bad for them?" However, there are a few main contributors that are worth mentioning.

First, food gives us too many short-term rewards. Food is delightful on many different levels, and people eat for a variety of reasons that don't involve eating to survive and keep healthy. For many of us, eating to stay alive is at best an afterthought when we think about eating, if it even comes up at all.

Second, there are usually no noticeable, immediate consequences to overeating. When we lose self-control in other aspects of life, there is usually an immediate consequence for failing to control our urges. If we choose to sleep late every day and miss work, we will lose our jobs. If we cheat on our spouses, we pay for it in divorce court. If we steal from a bank, we spend time in prison. But when it comes to eating, there is no Food Police, no matter how much it seems like there may be. Having an extra slice of pizza or two doesn't automatically put us in prison or start arguments. In fact, the opposite happens—it usually tastes pretty good and we get what seems to be positive reinforcement. It is only after months and years of eating like this that we gain too much weight and our bodies start to suffer.

When it comes to our basic behaviors such as eating, we often revert to the child within. If we are immediately punished for an action, we won't do it. If, on the other hand, we can "treat our-selves," and if it proves enjoyable without any immediate conse-quences, you can bet your bootstraps that many of us are going to do it again. I think this pretty much sums up the American obses-sion with food. With so many pleasurable activities forbidden or controlled, overeating is one of the few vices we can enjoy and not be immediately punished. In fact, in many ways, our culture encourages this. Restaurants serve larger and larger portions for less money, and all-you-can-eat buffets are commonplace. Eating con-tests are now a sport you can watch on TV.

After eating too much, most of us always think, "This is the last time I eat like this" or "I'll make up for this at a later time." I ask you: how many times have you lived up to that promise? We are a nation of procrastinators and optimists and this applies to our health, too. How many diets have you planned on starting "tomorrow"? The only problem is that tomorrow never seems to become today.

Some Healthy Reminders

So as we begin to look at a meal plan for weight and blood sugar control, we need to keep the following things in mind.

1. Overeating does come with a cost. It may not be immediate, but take one look at the average American waist size, coupled with our disturbing rates of diabetes, heart disease, and can-cer, and you soon realize the hidden cost of a poor diet.

2. Any healthy meal plan has to involve some self-control. I'm not saying you have to starve yourself and I'm not saying you can't enjoy food, but just as you cannot sleep late every morn-ing, just as you cannot pair off with everyone you meet, and just as you cannot rob a bank, you cannot eat whatever and whenever you want. When it comes to eating, self-control is just as important as all of the other daily urges we keep under control.

3. Finally, you will be required to exercise self-control on sever-al different levels and to many degrees. For example, if you have two beers a day, that's certainly better than six, but is it still good for your health? If you only eat fast food two days a week, but have it for breakfast, lunch, and dinner on those days, is it still okay? You need to use your common sense and avoid procrastinating. Ideally, none of us would ever eat fast food burgers. But if you eat it for two meals a day for five days

a week and cut down to just two meals in one week, I'd say you've made a lot of progress.

On the same note, eating habits such as snacking and grazing can be just as devastating to your health as the examples above. If you eat the ingredients of your meal while you're cooking it, you have to consider the effect that will have on your diet. Eating something just to keep yourself occupied while at work or at home adds up to unnecessary pounds. Little things in your meals can have a huge impact, too. That little extra pat of butter you put on your dinner roll can add up to a lot of extra calories over the course of several years. Why bother weighing yourself down for about a teaspoon of butter on a roll? I think it'd be a lot easier to skip that butter now than lose weight later in life.

It's Up to You

Losing weight, exercising, and taking care of your diabetes all require a great deal of self-control. When it comes to self-control, you are the only person who makes the decision whether you will follow through on losing weight or not. These are choices, and the road to better health means that you'll have to start making tough decisions that cause you to deny yourself instant gratification. You can do so, I believe, because you'll soon find out that the long-term benefits of these decisions far outweigh the short-term bliss of eating too much. Other words come to mind right now: discipline, willpower, and faith. You are capable of all of these things, and I believe that everyone has it within themselves to make the 1-2-3 Diabetes Diet work for them. Remember, if you lapse in self-control, you can always go back and start over right after that lapse. Giving up, however, only lets *you* down.

Chapter 8
Six Reasons Why Losing Weight Is So Hard

The difficulties of self-control are not the only factors making weight loss so hard. In addition to the psychological obstacles, there are a variety of physical and social roadblocks as well. Of the many out there, here are six big reasons losing weight is so hard.

#1 GOD MADE IT THAT WAY

Our bodies are designed to survive harsh conditions. When we were cavemen living in the wild, food was scarce. People could not farm effectively, and hunting was an unreliable source of food at best. Therefore, early humans who could retain as many extra calories as possible from their infrequent meals possessed an evolutionary advantage. When times got tough and no food was available, those humans who could save extra calories outlived those who could not retain calories. Of course, the way humans store extra calories is in the form of fat. Thus, the ability to store fat and slowly burn the calories it contains was a really helpful trait to have. Carrying a few extra pounds was the difference between surviving the winter and starving to death. If anything, evolution has hardwired your body to make dying as difficult as possible, so putting on weight is relatively easy and losing it is hard.

However, things are quite different in our modern lifestyles. Food is plentiful. Food is processed, produced, cooked, and manipulated in countless ways. Early humans had one way of getting from point A to point B—walking. What does this all add up to? Well, it means that early humans got a lot more exercise than we do and that they did not eat nearly as much food, especially high-calorie processed foods. Their eating and burning of calories were pretty close to equal (although they were usually eating fewer calories than they were burning), making for more or less healthy weights. Therefore, obesity and its related health problems were never really a consideration.

Q&A

Wait a minute. Based on evolution, it sounds like being obese or overweight is actually a good thing. Fat people are just prepared to survive disaster, right?

Well, yes and no. Being able to store energy in the form of fat and to burn it slowly is a good thing when food sources are scarce. However, most of us in the U.S. and other wealthy nations no longer have to worry about the availability of food. Early humans were hardly ever obese or overweight because they couldn't find and eat enough food to get that large. Plus, they were very physically active. This is no longer the case with the average American (though it does still apply in some parts of the world that are not as fortunate as ours). Being able to store a meal to last you a couple of days is a good thing when it may be your only meal for a while. But constantly carrying around a month's worth of calories (about 20 pounds of body weight) and not burning them is very hard on your body. The benefits of increased technology have made our lives much easier, but it has also come at a high price—in the form of health risks posed by excessive weight and lack of physical activity.

#2 FOOD TASTES SO DARN GOOD

Humans have five senses to explore and enjoy the world around them. While all of them are pleasant, taste can be a particularly powerful sense. As I just pointed out, eating and storing calories in the form of fat were originally helpful survival traits, so it is not surprising that the foods that have the most calories are often the tastiest. Fatty foods help us build up a large reserve of energy that may be helpful during harsh times, so they taste especially good. It is normal to like the taste of food, but if this enjoyment of tastes leads to overeating, then it can ultimately lead to weight gain.

#3 EATING IS A SOCIAL EVENT

Many of the social interactions and events in human culture revolve around food. When we celebrate, we eat. Holidays, birthdays, anniversaries, graduations, and promotions almost always involve dinners and parties filled with food and drink. For your birthday, you might get a buttery cake topped with sugary icing. Going out with friends is often as much about eating as it is socializing. Consider that most of the time, we go out to dinner or lunch with friends.

With all these opportunities to gorge going on around us, no wonder it is so easy to gain weight. After all, who wants to miss the party?

#4 WE EAT FOR REASONS OTHER THAN HUNGER

Some people eat because they are bored. Some eat because they are sad or worried. Many people eat just because the clock says that it is lunchtime. One key to weight loss is identifying some of these instances in your life. If you are eating for any reason other than hunger, you are eating and adding weight for no good reason.

#5 DIETING IS TOO MUCH WORK

Sure, dieting can be hard. But when you boil it down to its essentials, dieting is nothing more than thinking about what you are eating and making decisions. Is thought that hard? I personally believe everything important in life requires thought. It amazes me that people will spend hours of their day buying and caring for clothes, coordinating outfits, and grooming their appearance and yet not put any effort into choosing what and how they eat. Don't these activities both ultimately affect a person's appearance?

On the other hand, I don't think that monitoring your diet has to consume your entire life. Anything that controls every aspect of

An Addiction?

Some people eat because of complex psychological reasons. Patients with clinical depression or anxiety disorders sometimes use food to comfort themselves. Depressed people can often find temporary comfort in a gallon of ice cream. For people such as this, diet is more than an issue of watching what they eat. Food and eating help overcome issues in daily life and have become a way to cope with bigger issues. People with these problems should seek counseling or medication. I've seen several people lose tremendous amounts of weight once they treat their underlying depression.

Compulsive overeating often goes unnoticed because our culture supports eating. However, people who are compulsive overeaters often eat beyond the point where they are pleasantly full and their eating takes on an uncontrollable, frenzied pace. If this may be a possibility in your case, a good place to start would be to ask your doctor to refer you to a counselor or therapist. Thankfully, about 80% of compulsive overeaters can recover completely or make big steps forward with proper professional help.

your life will eventually lead you to reject it. That's not what we want. A well-planned diet will find a happy middle ground, but ultimately any lifestyle change (including your diet) will require some effort.

#6 IT FEELS BAD TO DIET

Most diets ask you to give up too much. In these cases, you always feel hungry and never get to eat what tastes good. In most diets, the costs required to lose weight defeat the benefits, setting up dieters for failure. Everyone would lose weight if they decided to eat a steady diet of salad greens without dressing or anything else, but no one would stick with such a diet because it requires too much sacrifice. It doesn't have to be this way. In my mind, the ideal diet, when combined with exercise, should do the following:

1. Help you lose weight.
2. Allow you to eat throughout the day and not feel hungry.
3. Allow you splurge at times, enjoy tasty food, and keep up the lifestyle you want.
4. Provide total nutrition and promote fitness.
5. Not be complicated or difficult to follow.

Does that sound like too much of a sacrifice? Too much work? No, you won't be able to eat pizza and burgers all day long, but you won't be eating pea-sized portions of rabbit food either. Instead, you'll be eating just the right amount.

Chapter 9
Six Reasons Why
You Should Lose Weight

So we've covered some of the reasons dieting is no easy task and this is important. Recognizing potential pitfalls is always the best way to develop a strategy. Now it's time to focus on the upside of dieting. Use these six reasons as motivation to get started and stick with it.

#1 YOU'LL LOOK BETTER

Do you remember the days when you were thinner? Do you remember the outfits that you used to wear? Do you remember what you looked like in the mirror? If you lose weight, that could be you again.

#2 YOU'LL FEEL BETTER

When people like how they look, they feel better about themselves and the world. Yet, the differences go further than skin deep. I'd bet you wouldn't like to carry around a 50-pound barbell all the time; by the end of the day, you would feel tired and sore. Yet when you're 50 pounds overweight, this is exactly what you are doing. This is why obese people often suffer from fatigue, moodiness, and insomnia. Aside from the very real health risks connected to obesity, these conditions can physically and emotionally drain a person on a daily basis.

Losing weight not only makes you lighter, but it can also give you energy, improve your heart and respiratory function, and take the stress off your joints. I've never seen patients as happy as when they have lost some weight. When you feel better and accomplish something as difficult as losing weight, you become encouraged to take further steps to feel even better.

#3 LOSING WEIGHT CAN PREVENT OR DELAY TYPE 2 DIABETES

A recent clinical study, the Diabetes Prevention Program, looked at people who were at risk for the development of type 2 diabetes due to obesity. The study divided the subjects into three treatment groups. The first followed a program of diet and exercise, the second took an oral diabetes pill called metformin, and the third took a placebo pill. Those who increased their physical activity (30 minutes a day for five days a week) and lost modest amounts of weight (about 10–15 pounds, or 7% of their total body weight) avoided developing diabetes or took longer to develop the disease. In fact, the group that simply followed the diet-and-exercise treatment had the best results over the three years of the study.

#4 YOUR BLOOD SUGAR WILL PROBABLY IMPROVE

When people start taking medication for diabetes, they often ask me if they will ever be able to stop it. Unfortunately, in many cases, especially if the person is very insulin resistant or has advanced diabetes, this may realistically never happen. Early in the disease, however, you may have a chance to reverse the initial stages of diabetes. For many people, modest to moderate weight loss can reduce insulin resistance enough to make a noticeable difference. I have seen several people (particularly those who seriously improved their diet and exercised hard) who have lost weight and have been able to cut back or stop their diabetes medications altogether. For most people with type 2 diabetes, every pound lost can lead to improved blood sugar control and may even save you some money on medication costs.

#5 YOUR OVERALL HEALTH WILL IMPROVE

As we have seen, obesity is linked to other health risks besides diabetes, including elevated cholesterol and hypertension. Instead of waiting for a major heart attack or stroke, look at your waist size, get serious about your health, and get the weight off.

#6 YOU WILL LIVE LONGER

Obesity is a major cause of death in the United States. Multiple studies have shown that there is a direct link between high BMI and mortality. Obese people die younger and more frequently from almost every type of disorder, including heart disease and cancer. For many obese patients, losing weight is ultimately the key to improved health and a longer, happier life.

The Bottom Line on Obesity

As much as we hate to think about it, all of us eventually die, no matter how many pills we take. If you are obese, you will also die, but odds are that you'll die at a younger age or suffer from years of poor health. This thought causes a lot of people to resign themselves to a gloomy, fatalistic approach. "I'm going to die someday anyway, so what's the point?" Whether or not someone actually believes this, it ignores a pretty big point: You are not the only one who cares whether or not you're alive. Perhaps losing weight and getting your diabetes under control could add years to your life, enough to get a chance to see your children and grandchildren grow up, to spend that much more time with your family and those who care for you. If all it would take is losing some weight, how could you not at least try? It's certainly not easy, but the benefits of losing weight are much greater than the costs.

SECTION HIGHLIGHTS
A Brief Summary of Important Points
Discussed in this Section

1. The first step in the 1-2-3 Diabetes Diet is to think about eating. This is tough and often new to many people. Thinking about eating can be broken down into three questions:

   - How do you eat? This includes when you eat, where you eat, and what other things you do while you eat.
   - What do you eat? Most of us know what we should be eating. Unfortunately, we often ignore this information.
   - How much do you eat? Portion sizes have grown out of control in this country. Just eating smaller servings of the things we like is the biggest thing we can do to lose weight.

2. The key to maintaining a healthy diet is self-control. You know (probably even without reading this book) what you need to do to stay healthy. However, employing self-control in situations where there are no immediate consequences is very, very difficult. If something is truly important, we will give it the time it requires. Your health should always be this important. Just thinking a little bit more about eating will start to have results.

3. In addition to the difficulty of self-control, here is why it's hard to lose weight:

   - People are genetically built to hold onto fat for survival.
   - Food just tastes so good.
   - Many of our social events revolve around eating.
   - We eat for reasons other than hunger.
   - Dieting feels bad.

4. Here's why going through all of that hard work is worth it:

   - You'll look better.
   - You'll feel better, emotionally and physically.
   - Losing weight can prevent or delay developing type 2 diabetes.
   - Less weight can improve your blood sugar levels.
   - Your overall health will improve.
   - You'll live longer.

Step Two:
Make Healthy Changes

Chapter 10
Weight Loss: As Simple as 1-2-3

By now, it should be pretty apparent that a healthy weight is very important to proper diabetes management. We have also just explored the reasons why losing weight is so hard. All the details aside, it boils down to this: Americans, both with and without diabetes, eat more than they should and, at the same time, eat more of the wrong foods than they should.

There are many theories about weight loss, and I'm sure most of you have tried many of them. The problem is that most are fad diets or quick-fix programs (take a magic pill and you'll lose weight with no effort! Eat nothing but bacon and mustard and the pounds will melt away!) that focus on unrealistic eating habits. These unrealistic programs become impossible to maintain for a long time. Thus, you might lose a few pounds in the beginning of a low-carb diet, but it's impossible to stick with it for a long time and eventually you gain back the weight. You can only eat hamburgers without buns for so long. These fad diets can be especially rough on people with diabetes because these diets often worsen blood sugar control.

In addition, diets that rely exclusively on eating only one type of food do not provide nutritional balance and are ultimately unhealthy. For example, high-fat diets can result in high cholesterol levels and increased risk of cancer. On the same note, a poorly planned vegetarian diet can result in low levels of protein and calcium, which can lead to muscle loss and poor bone health. If you have diabetes, you need to maintain a healthy mix of nutrients in order to stay medically fit.

How then does a person lose weight and keep it off? The answer lies in learning some simple facts about nutrition, making appropriate changes to your eating patterns, and sticking to these changes for life. Weight loss will require some work, but in the end should easily fit into any person's lifestyle. Your diet should and can be as much work as deciding what to wear for a day.

Weight loss basically relies on the balance of calories coming in versus the calories being burned. If you burn more calories than you eat, then fat will get broken down and you *have* to lose weight. This can be accomplished by either burning more calories than you currently are or by eating fewer calories. On the other hand, if you eat more calories than you burn, you will gain weight. When you look at it this way, a weight-loss meal plan is as simple as:

1. Choosing an appropriate number of calories to eat in a day that, when combined with a healthy physical activity level, will result in weight loss (starving yourself to lose weight while avoiding exercise is both dangerous and unwise).
2. Making a plan that divides all of these calories into meals throughout the day.
3. Sticking to that plan.

This looks so simple that it seems almost too ridiculous to work. If this is all there is to it, why isn't everyone doing this?

As simple as this plan looks on paper, putting this into practice is more complicated than it first appears. There are many pitfalls and traps along the way, not the least of which is our huge appetite for high-calorie foods. You will be constantly tempted along the way by junk food in the grocery store, the fast-food joints that are everywhere (offering speedy service and inexpensive food), and other people eating what you wish you could be eating. Remember how I keep mentioning self-control? This is where it's put to the test.

But this is about more than just losing weight. We also need to consider the special needs that come along with diabetes. You have a further concern in that your diet needs to produce consistent blood sugar levels throughout the day. In addition, a good diabetes diet needs to address cholesterol and blood pressure. The diet I propose does all of this and more. If done correctly, my 1-2-3 Diabetes Diet should:

1. Keep a person at a stable, healthy weight
2. Maintain a constant, target-range blood sugar
3. Provide nutritional balance
4. Fit into a simple fulfilling meal plan

Can this plan work? It certainly can, I've seen it work time and time again with the patients in my clinic. Now it's time to let it work for you, and I'll tell you how.

Chapter 11
Add It Up: Calorie Counting

The first step to weight loss is learning to count calories. As you begin to keep your food diary, you're going to need to know how many calories you're currently eating so that you can see where to make adjustments. As you go along, you'll use calorie counting to figure out how to build a meal plan that will work for you and to help you make sure you're sticking to your plan. We'll talk more about analyzing your food diary, making adjustments, and creating your meal plan in the rest of this section. Right now, let's discuss how to keep track of the calories you eat.

SIMPLE MATH

As I mentioned, the amount of food you eat has to match the number of calories you burn in a day or you'll gain weight. It's simple math: if you eat more calories than you burn, the leftovers are stored as fat. On the other hand, if you burn more calories than you eat, then the fat burns off and you lose some weight. This is the key to successful, long-term weight loss. The calorie count total for a day consists of two practical parts:

1. *Calorie content.* As you already know, every morsel of food has a number of calories. Some foods, like those with a lot of fat, have more calories than others do, even though the serving size may be the same. I bet you knew that, too. To get even more scientific, each gram of fat in a food contains 9 calories. On the other hand, each gram of carbohydrate or protein has only 4 calories. Therefore, a slice of pepperoni pizza with 9 grams of fat, 11 grams of protein, and 28 grams of carbohydrates has 237 calories (9 × 9 = 81 fat calories, 11 × 4 = 44 pro-

tein calories, and 28 × 4 = 112 carbohydrate calories, which totals 81 + 44 + 112 = 237 calories).

2. *Portion size.* Your daily calorie count is the total number of calories for every morsel of food that you consume in a given day. If you have five slices of the above pizza, that's 1,185 calories (5 slices = 237 + 237 + 237 + 237 + 237). If you have a Calorie Ceiling of 1,800 calories a day (we'll determine your Calorie Ceiling in just a bit), then you only have 615 calories left for your remaining meals and snacks for the day. That's not much, so you can probably see why even holding off on one slice of pizza may be a good idea.

How Is This Simple?

At this point, you may be scratching your head. If you are like many people, you don't see food in terms of calories. When you're looking at a taco with beef and cheese, you don't see 14 grams of carbohydrate, 14 grams of fat, and 9 grams of protein and add it up to about 218 calories. What about the soda you're drinking with the taco? You'll starve to death before you finish doing all that math. Instead, you probably see one delicious little taco and wish you could have more than one.

Some diet authors assume that adding up calories is too complex and too much trouble for the average person on the go. I agree. Maybe if you had a calorimeter (a device that measures the calorie content of food) and a calculator around at every meal, you could do this. But most of the time, a meal plan that requires you to accurately calculate calories from scratch isn't going to last very long. However, it is very important that you know the calorie count of the food you eat in a day if you want to lose weight. No matter what diet you are on, if you eat more calories than you burn, you will gain weight. How can you expect to lose weight if you don't have some idea of what you are putting into your body?

In order to do this, calorie counting has to be easy. Accurately measuring every single calorie in your sandwich might be unrealistic, but it's not that hard to learn how to "guestimate" the number of calories your food contains. A person usually eats only a few different types of foods, so once you start to get an understanding of the calorie contents of your favorite foods, it isn't too hard to start tracking the calories you are consuming. It doesn't have to be perfect; ballpark figures are better than nothing at all. The bottom line is that ignoring how many calories you're eating in a day clearly isn't the path to lifelong weight loss.

Your Calorie Counting Toolbox

It's always nice to have a helping hand for any tough endeavor. Fortunately, a number of tools exist to make calorie counting easier. A few of the most common include:

1. **Guidebooks.** You've seen these little books in grocery store lines. They list the nutrition contents of many foods you find in restaurants and grocery stores, including the foods you make at home. These can provide the most information for you, but also require the most effort. The American Diabetes Association's *Guide to Healthy Restaurant Eating*, 3rd Edition, and *Diabetes Carbohydrate and Fat Gram Guide*, 3rd Edition, are very handy examples of such books.

2. **Nutrition Facts Labels.** The Nutrition Facts Label is the rectangular white box with nutrition information you see on every package of food. This can be your best friend when it comes to counting calories. The key to using the Nutrition Facts is making sure you count how many actual servings of food you are eating. Let's say you buy a 12-ounce bag of potato chips. The serving size listed on the bag is 3 ounces—which means there are four servings in the bag—and there are 120 calories in a serving. If you eat the whole bag, you need to count the calories for four servings (480 calories), not just one.

Nutrition Facts		
Serving Size 1 cup (228g)		
Servings Per Container 2		
Amount Per Serving		
Calories 260		Calories from Fat 120
		% Daily Value*
Total Fat 13g		**20%**
Saturated Fat 5g		**25%**
Trans Fat 2g		
Cholesterol 30mg		**10%**
Sodium 660mg		**28%**
Total Carbohydrate 31g		**10%**
Dietary Fiber 0g		**0%**
Sugars 5g		
Protein 5g		
Vitamin A 4%	•	Vitamin C 2%
Calcium 15%	•	Iron 4%

* Percent Daily Values are based on a 2,000 calorie diet. Your Daily Values may be higher or lower depending on your calorie needs.

	Calories:	2,000	2,500
Total Fat	Less than	65g	80g
Sat Fat	Less than	20g	25g
Cholesterol	Less than	300mg	300mg
Sodium	Less than	2,400mg	2,400mg
Total Carbohydrate		300g	375mg
Dietary Fiber		25g	30g

Calories per gram:
Fat 9 • Carbohydrate 4 • Protein 4

3. **Research.** Many of the restaurants we visit post the nutrition information for their menu items on their website or make it available on their menus or by request. Finding this data (and reading the fine print: sometimes the nutrition information provided doesn't include sauces that normally come with the food) can make it easy to choose healthy options wherever you go out to eat.

The thing to keep in mind when choosing a method of counting calories is ease of use. It can be very handy to have a guide nearby, so when you eat at your favorite restaurant and order something from the menu, you can find out exactly how many calories you just ate, as well as the other nutritional content. Eventually, you will probably want to be able to simply look at a food item and estimate its nutritional and caloric value. That will come in time, as you become more experienced in working with your diet. No one knows the alphabet the second they're born; they have to learn it. Think of calorie counting the same way and practice, practice, practice.

Chapter 12
Reading Your Food Diary

In Chapter 4, I talked about the importance of keeping a food diary. Maybe you've already started jotting down your eating habits, maybe you plan to start doing so soon. Either way, this is an important step in your weight-loss program. Using the calorie counting tools I discussed in Chapter 11 should help you estimate how many calories you are currently eating, in addition to the other information you should be tracking. Now we're going to discuss how you can use this information to make healthy changes.

ANALYZING YOUR EATING INFORMATION

Reading your food diary can be a sobering experience. After all, facing you will be at least a week's worth of eating habits and a log of every piece of food you've put in your mouth. On paper, this can seem like a lot. But as disheartening as this can be, it may be just the wake-up call you need. Think of it this way: everything written on the pages of your food diary has led to you being overweight and, therefore, understanding your food diary is the key to losing weight in the future.

I know getting to this step may be a difficult process, but you're not alone. One of the more common complaints about food diaries is that it takes too much time to keep up with it. This is certainly true. Finding time in our busy schedules for any additional activity is hard. The easiest way to conquer this problem when keeping your food diary is to make it a priority. Much of the 1-2-3 Diabetes Diet (and any other successful weight-loss program) relies on self-motivation. The motivation it takes to keep your food diary is the same motivation you'll need to continue losing weight. If you have a few gaps in your diary, a few skipped days, don't give up. Just pick up where you left off and leave the skipped days empty. Just because your food diary isn't a complete log of seven consecutive days doesn't mean that it's useless.

Look Objectively

An important strategy to follow when interpreting your food diary is to look at it with an objective point of view. Many people are tempted upon first glance to make excuses for themselves or try to "explain away" why or what they ate at that particular moment. As strong as this temptation may be, do your best to resist. Making excuses for your eating patterns will keep you from making changes. The easiest way to approach this is to imagine that you're looking at the food diary of another person and examine it like a puzzle. If this were a co-worker's food diary, what changes would you recommend?

Find Patterns

Finding patterns often proves to be the easiest way to solve a puzzle. Your food diary is no different. Identifying patterns will help locate those elusive eating habits that I've been talking about. Often just asking yourself questions about the information in front of you will help uncover patterns that you can change. Here is a list of possible questions.

- Which meal contains the highest number of calories on average?
- How many snacks do I have in a day?
- How many calories are in my snacks? Do they match a normal meal?
- What kind of foods do I normally eat in a day?
- How large are my servings?
- Am I eating any vegetables? Any fruit?
- What foods do I eat with too much fat?
- How often do I eat out in a week? In a day? Why? Am I too busy or is it due to social events?
- What errands or tasks do I have on days when my eating habits are wildly different?
- When I eat on the run (such as hitting the drive-through window or stopping at the mall while driving home), what kinds of foods do I eat?
- What is my general mood when I eat? Are there patterns between what I eat and my emotions?
- In general, how hungry am I when I eat? How does this compare to the amount of food I'm eating in a given meal?

When you answer these questions, look to see if the same answer applies day after day. Look for common associations between what, when, and how you are eating. For example, if you're eating an afternoon snack of about 1,000 calories Monday through Friday, that's an eating habit you've just identified. If you find that you're eating fast food for three meals on days when you have tons of errands to run, then you can try to change that pattern. Are the foods you eat high in fat but low in other nutrients? You can change that. If you find that you're eating a lot of food when you're only moderately hungry, then perhaps you can address this issue.

Avoid broad generalities and focus on specifics. The examples above are specific. General patterns will not direct you toward anything you can change. You can avoid this (and make reading your food diary easier) by asking specific questions much like those above. Avoid general questions like:

- Why am I fat?
- What is wrong with me?
- Am I eating too many calories in a day?

These questions don't lead you to answers. Instead, they may make you feel bad about yourself and that doesn't lead to solutions to problems. You need to stay focused. Avoid interrogating yourself like this. More broad patterns include:

- I eat too much.
- I'm too busy to worry about what I eat.
- I eat all of the time.

Generic patterns such as these won't point you toward a solution. If you simply say, "I eat too much," then where do you cut out some of that extra food? It's hard to pinpoint a solution when you can't find the problem. If you do eat too much, then *when* do you eat too much? Which meals? What are you eating? Better yet, *where* in your diet can you eat less food?

Don't feel that you have to find every single pattern in your food diary. This is a work in progress, so if you only find two or three issues, that's fine. As you move further along in your weight-loss program, you'll have more opportunities to look closely at your food diary and unearth further areas you can change. In addition, as you gain more experience in controlling your diet and monitoring your eating habits, you'll have an easier time looking closely at your eating habits.

As you look for eating patterns, jot them down on a piece of paper so you don't forget them. Doing this will also keep you from finding the same pattern and just saying it in different ways (for example, "I eat when I am not hungry" and "I eat meals when I don't need to"). Try to find one or two specific patterns from your food diary—starting small will be the key to losing weight over time.

Behavioral Triggers

As you examine your food diary and try to identify patterns, one of the things you'll need to look for are *behavioral triggers*. These are actions or situations that can lead you to overeat. Examples include coming home from work, watching TV, getting ready for bed, or high-stress situations. Many times, these situations in our daily routine become so associated with eating that they cause us to crave food without us realizing it. Does turning on the TV suddenly compel you to grab a bag of chips from the kitchen? When things are stressful at work, do you start munching on snacks without realizing it? These situations are behavioral triggers and breaking them can be hard.

Fighting behavioral triggers is a two-step process. The first step is recognizing them. The second is replacing them with healthy triggers. Instead of grabbing that bag of chips when you turn on the TV, do some light exercise while you're watching the five o'clock news. After a while, you'll come to associate watching the news with exercise. Instead of mindlessly eating chocolate when you're stressed, turn this into an opportunity to take a brief walk and clear your head.

You can also create new behavioral triggers and use them to your advantage. For example, if you're still hungry at the end of your more sensibly sized meals, eat a light, healthy dessert such as yogurt or a fruit cup after you're done with your dinner. Then use this activity as a trigger to signify you're done eating. After a while, your body and mind will learn to recognize this healthy dessert as the end of your meal and your craving for more food will fade away.

Changing Patterns One at a Time

By reading and assessing your food diary, you may have decided that you need to change many things, such as eating less fried food, not skipping breakfast every day, and having fewer snacks. However, don't try to make all of these changes in one day. You formed your eating habits over years, so changing them won't happen immediately. Of the many habits we have, eating habits are particularly difficult to change. This is why you need to set goals one at a time.

How do you choose which habit to change first? Choose one that you feel you can change easily. If you successfully change one habit, you're more likely to tackle the next. An easy change may be switching to a healthier food for nighttime snacks or choosing non-fat milk over whole milk. A more difficult change would be cutting out every snack throughout the day.

Key Points for Realistic Goals

Your new eating habit goals should

- be realistic
- be easy to achieve
- be specific
- have a short time frame

Realistic goals means there's a lower possibility of failure. If goals are specific, you know what to do to achieve them. A short time frame lets you track how well you are doing in following through on these goals.

Example

You notice that you get a fast-food breakfast during the workweek, which is generally a sausage biscuit and hash browns. This breakfast is filled with many unnecessary calories and puts too much fat and cholesterol in your diet. You decide that this is an easy place to begin changing your diet.

Therefore, for the next two months (*short time frame*), two days each week (*specific*), you will eat one of these two healthier breakfasts: 1) an English muffin with jelly and a small banana or 2) half of a bagel with light cream cheese and an orange (*realistic* and *easy to achieve*).

Look at your recent food records or think about what you eat day in and day out. Make your goals easy to reach. Keep your goals handy, so you can see them frequently—in your calendar, on the refrigerator, or on your night table. At the end of the time frame you set, answer these questions:

- Did I meet my goals?
- How much so? Was it 60% of the time? 80%?
- If not, why not? Were they unrealistic?
- Was the time frame too long?

If you did not meet your goals, then make them easier to accomplish or choose another one that you can achieve. If you met your goals, pat yourself on the back!

Remember, practicing a new habit day after day and month after month makes it become a part of you. For example, if you always remember to stick a piece of fruit in your briefcase or lunchbox before you leave home in the morning and eat it during the afternoon, then you'll notice if you forget that fruit in the morning. It's become habit. If you make it a habit to avoid croutons on your salads at lunch, eventually you'll forget to think about putting them on your salad. If you start taking walks after lunch at work, after a while, you'll notice if you don't get that brief after-lunch walk on a normal workday.

Chapter 13
Creating Your Calorie Ceiling

So now you know a bit about calorie counting and you've studied your food diary to find patterns and see where you can make adjustments. The next step is to decide on a Calorie Ceiling for your day. The adjustments you make to your eating patterns should put you within your Calorie Ceiling. There has to be a limit on the amount of food you eat if you want to lose weight and maintain your blood sugars. Despite all of the hype surrounding quick-and-easy diets, if there isn't any form of calorie control, then losing weight and keeping it off is impossible. So how do you decide on a Calorie Ceiling?

WHERE TO START?

If you are a man, start with a Calorie Ceiling of about 2,000 calories a day. If you are a woman, begin with about 1,800 calories a day. If you are a particularly large man, maybe you could start at about 2,200 calories, but no more than that. If you are a particularly small woman, you could start at about 1,600 calories a day. Do not go below 1,200 calories a day without discussing this with your physician or dietitian.

This may seem a little random, as if I pulled the numbers out of thin air. In fact, these Calorie Ceilings are modeled after the calorie-restricted diet most physicians would recommend to their patients. The way I view things, you need to start somewhere; adjustments to your Calorie Ceiling can come later depending on your needs. After all, do people run marathons if they haven't run over a mile in months? No way! They train and make additions to their running routine over time. This is how you should view your initial Calorie Ceiling: a good place to start.

I'll bet that for many of you, the Calorie Ceilings we are discussing (1,200–2,400 calories a day) are well below the number of calories you are currently eating in a day. Typically, starting with a Calorie Ceiling level of 1,600–2,000 calories a day will satisfy most appetites, lead to gradual weight loss, and lead to better blood sugar control. Keeping your appetite satisfied will be one of the more important parts of selecting your Calorie Ceiling. We eat too much food these days, but starving yourself is no good either. If you feel severely deprived of food, you'll likely lapse and binge. You don't want that. You want a manageable amount of calories going in, but not so many that you can't possibly burn them off through exercise.

In terms of people with diabetes, the other important aspect of the Calorie Ceiling concept is that diabetes is best treated when a person eats the same amount of calories day to day. Splurging and starving make proper glucose control very difficult. In addition, diabetes pills and insulin work best with a stable diet. You can help avoid very high or very low blood glucose levels by eating at or near the same Calorie Ceiling every day and spreading your calories throughout the day in a consistent fashion. Remember, though, that the nutrient content of your meals will have a greater effect on your blood sugar levels than pure calorie content. You can really improve your diabetes care later, when you are ready for carbohydrate counting.

Keep in mind that your Calorie Ceiling isn't a fixed amount that you have to live with for the rest of your life. You should try to stick with your beginning Calorie Ceiling for at least a week and monitor your progress. Start weighing yourself. Get used to eating a healthier diet. Get used to not eating as much food. This will take some training for your body, and it takes time. When you finish a meal, sit back and wait awhile, and see if you're still hungry. If you are, eat a little bit more, but not enough to add up to another full serving. You will find that over time, your body will become used to the amount of food you eat daily. Just as your body was used to your old diet, your body will become used to your new diet and you will feel satisfied from your healthier meal.

After you've tried things for a little while, adjust your Calorie Ceiling each day depending on what you want to achieve. Not losing weight fast enough? Cut back your Calorie Ceiling by 100 or 200 calories a day. Are you losing a good amount of weight but always hungry? Add 200 calories a day to your Calorie Ceiling. Keep in mind that since you'll be eating less food than normal, you *will be hungrier than normal at first.* This is just natural. However, if you stick with it, your body will quickly adjust to the sensible servings you're now eating. As you can see, it won't matter what your starting Calorie Ceiling is because you will be adjusting it to your specific needs over time.

A Warning

It is not healthy to starve yourself to lose weight, and it's downright dangerous if you have diabetes. If you're not losing weight fast enough, there are healthy ways to boost your metabolism and burn calories. Instead of starving yourself and trying to eat only 500 calories, eat a healthy amount of food and increase your exercise level. We'll talk more about exercise in Chapter 21.

CALCULATING A SPECIFIC CALORIE CEILING

So you've looked at the beginning Calorie Ceilings I mentioned above but you feel they may not apply to you. You want a more exact Calorie Ceiling tailored to you. Here's an easy way to approach setting your own specific Calorie Ceiling. Just grab a calculator and fill out the blanks below.

To maintain your current weight (not lose or gain any pounds):
Your weight _____ × 11 = _____ current calories.

To lose 1 pound a week:
current calories (from above) _____ – 500 = _____ calories per day.

To lose 2 pounds a week:
current calories (from above) ____ – 1,000 = _____ calories per day.

Remember to start slow and try to lose one pound a week. Doing too much in the beginning can be too much of a shock to your system. Shooting for two pounds a week may be too difficult a goal for most people in the beginning because you'll be eating a lot less food than you are used to. I recommend starting at one pound a week and using exercise to burn calories. If you've filled this out, you've probably found that the Calorie Ceilings I mentioned earlier are close to the Calorie Ceilings you're getting from this formula.

To make things a little more concrete, let's use an example. Say we have a guy named Joe who has just been diagnosed with diabetes and needs to lose some weight. Right now, Joe weighs 220 pounds. Using the formula above, Joe figures:

To maintain his weight:
220 × 11 = 2,420 current calories.

To lose 1 pound a week:
2,420 – 500 = 1,920 calories a day.

To lose 2 pounds a week:
2,420 – 1,000 = 1,420 calories a day.

See? It's not too different from the beginning Calorie Ceilings I estimated above. This formula also shows you to what extent you need to cut down your calorie intake to lose weight rapidly—it's a lot. Be patient. Don't try to do too much all at once. This is a marathon, not a sprint. Healthy weight loss takes time.

Two Possible Calorie Ceiling Pitfalls

1. If you are eating at a Calorie Ceiling that is causing gradual weight loss, but are absolutely starving all the time, see Chapter 23. Most likely, you are fighting hunger, but your Calorie Ceiling is working.

2. If you've cut your Calorie Ceiling way back and are still not losing weight, you may need extra help. A visit with a registered dietitian may help (see Chapter 29) or you can look for support in the resources listed in the Appendix.

Chapter 14
A Short Checklist

Y ou may be feeling a bit overwhelmed at this point in the book given all of the information that we have covered. Let's take a step back and make a checklist of the things you need to do to get this far in the 1-2-3 Diabetes Diet. Remember earlier in the book when I told you that starting a healthy diet may require a lot of thinking? This is where it becomes apparent. Never fear. After a little while a sensible, personal diet like this one will become a part of your life that you hardly ever have to think about.

 Begin a food diary.

A food diary will help you find out more about your eating habits, serving sizes, and what kinds of foods you're eating. A food diary will help you figure out how you eat, how much you eat, and what you eat. You should spend at least a week or two keeping your food diary.

Figure out how many calories you're eating in a day.

With the help of calorie-counting tools, your food diary will also show you how many calories you're eating every day. It will show you how many calories you'll have to cut out of your diet in order to lose weight. The number of calories you're consuming in a day will tie closely to the changes you need to make for portion control.

✓ *Figure out if you have eating habits that you should take care of.*

After you've spent some time keeping up with your food diary, you should look at it and try to find patterns. Look for eating habits that lead you to gain weight and start working on changing them. Your eating habits can have an effect on portion control.

✓ *Look at the types of foods you're eating in a day.*

The types of foods you're eating are closely tied to your calorie intake. Remember that fatty foods contain more calories than others, so you should definitely try to cut down on those. Portion control will help you cut down on these foods and still enjoy them in moderation.

✓ *Set a Calorie Ceiling.*

Your Calorie Ceiling is the starting point you're going to set in order to begin weight loss. You need to start somewhere. The general standard is 2,000 calories a day for men and 1,800 calories a day for women. This is probably far lower than the normal amount of calories you're currently eating per day.

✓ *Adjust your Calorie Ceiling to fit your needs and goals.*

You can gradually change your Calorie Ceiling in 100- or 200-calorie increments. If you're always hungry, add a small amount of calories and try that for a week. See what happens. If anything, you should be trying to cut out calories from your diet, so be careful before you start adding more and more calories to your diet; otherwise, you'll make no progress. Remember, weight loss takes time—it's not instant—so give your Calorie Ceiling a chance and watch the results. Of course, you have to follow the next step before you can tell if you'll need to make changes to your Calorie Ceiling.

✓ *Next step: Fit your Calorie Ceiling into a daily meal plan.*

Now that you've figured out where you need to make changes in your eating patterns (the total of your eating habits, what you eat, and how much you eat) and set a Calorie Ceiling, we're going to look at how to make this work in a practical situation.

Chapter 15

Spreading the Wealth:
Your Daily Meal Plan

Okay, so you have this Calorie Ceiling, but now what do you do with it? The answer is simple, you're going to take the number of calories you have for a given day and divide it into separate meals and snacks. This is very important because you have to eat regular meals to regulate your blood glucose levels. Spacing regular meals throughout the day also can prevent hunger and binging. By eating about every four to five hours, you keep your brain fueled, so you think better, and your metabolism keeps going. If you go for long periods without eating, your body goes into conservation mode to prevent starvation. What you're creating is called a meal plan, and many people with diabetes use meal plans to control their weight and blood glucose numbers.

THE 1-2-3 DIABETES DIET APPROACH

Unlike some meal plans, the 1-2-3 Diabetes Diet does not use exchange values for the foods you eat. Using exchange values is another meal plan system people with diabetes use to monitor their food intake. Exchange values give you a certain number of servings, or exchanges, of different kinds of foods over the course of a day. You can exchange these servings with other foods to maintain a healthy diet throughout the day. Though they are very helpful, exchange values can become complicated for some people. For them, exchanges don't seem to relate to how they eat or how they view food. That's why the 1-2-3 Diabetes Diet uses Calorie Ceilings instead of exchanges, because I feel counting calories and having a Calorie Ceiling is a lot like budgeting money, and that's something everyone seems to understand.

One thing to keep in mind is to make sure you're eating foods from many of the different food groups. Look back at the new food pyramid on page 51. You should aim to include enough foods in your meal plan to match the proportions displayed in the food pyramid. Doing this and watching your calorie intake at the same time will help you get all of your nutrients without gaining weight. Meal plans can take a little work, but after a while, you'll see that they're not so difficult to maintain. Losing weight will rely a lot on a successful meal plan, so let's look at what you should consider when putting together your meal plan.

Perfection Is Not the Goal

In a perfect world, we wouldn't need to follow a meal plan to lose weight and care for our diabetes. We'd all eat perfectly nutritious meals in the right amounts and get enough exercise to keep ourselves lean, fit, and healthy. But we hardly live in a perfect world. This is the real world, so your meal plan should be realistic as well. Striving for perfection is great in most cases, but not when it sets you up for failure. Small steps are the key to successful weight loss, not impossible goals.

Here's an example of what I mean. In a perfect world, your 1-2-3 Diabetes Diet meal plan would be flawless. You would pick the exact right Calorie Ceiling to lose weight healthily, about one pound a week. You would spread your calories throughout the day, perfectly timed with your medications and activities, and this meal plan would not change from day to day. Every meal would consist of a stable number of calories, and you would never splurge. Your blood sugar would always be right on target, you would never have hyperglycemia or hypoglycemia, and you would ever have to see a dietitian or doctor again.

Perhaps there's someone out there who can follow this routine perfectly. Most of you, though, see several problems with this perfect meal plan. Where's the time in this perfect meal plan to run errands after work? How do you find time to go to work in the first place? What about special events? Even more, it sounds boring eating the same meals every day. I wouldn't expect anyone to keep up with this strict regimen. It's okay to be human.

What you do need to realize, however, is that you can eat about the same number of calories every day and still have a great deal of diversity in the foods you eat. Meal planning allows for this, and even though you may occasionally go over your Calorie Ceiling, after a little bit of practice, you'll know enough to consistently keep close to it.

WHAT'S IN A MEAL PLAN?

By now you have a pretty good idea what your eating habits are from the food diary you've kept. You know how you eat, what you eat, and how much you eat. You also probably have a good idea of how the calories you eat balance with the calories you burn. Keep in mind that when you start eating fewer calories, you're also going to be taking in fewer nutrients, so paying close attention to what foods you are eating becomes more and more important. I've also shown you the new USDA food pyramid, which points out that you should do the following if you're striving to eat healthily. To review:

- About one-fifth of your foods should be grains, preferably whole grains.
- Eat more fruits; no one ever eats enough fruit.
- Mom was right; you need to eat your vegetables. Make sure you add some diversity to the vegetables you're eating, too. There's more out there than broccoli, peas, carrots, and corn.
- Don't eat as much meat. Meat is definitely an important part of a healthy diet because you get some key nutrients from it. However, Americans eat too much meat—to the point that it is unhealthy.
- The food pyramid emphasizes milk and dairy, but I suggest choosing nonfat or fat-free versions.
- Finally, make as many efforts as possible to cut down your intake of fats and oils. You can see that the food pyramid has a tiny sliver for these foods, and your meal plan should represent this as well.

When you create your own meal plan, you have to take all of these factors into account. You've spent a lot of time on analyzing yourself, and now it's time to put all of that hard-earned knowledge to use. Follow these simple steps to create your personal meal plan.

BUILDING YOUR MEAL PLAN IN TWO STEPS

1. Pick an ideal Calorie Ceiling. Remember that you are going to adjust your Calorie Ceiling as your situation changes. For starters, just pick a Calorie Ceiling that will start you down the path to modest weight loss. Don't shoot for the moon on your first Calorie Ceiling. If you're eating 3,000 calories a day right now and you set your Calorie Ceiling at 1,800 calories a day, what do you think will happen? You will probably fail. Aim for a Calorie Ceiling that is practical and achievable. If you're eating 3,000 calories a day, maybe 2,500 will work to begin with. As you get used to that level, you can lower it further. Remember, your goal in having a Calorie Ceiling is to lose weight and keep it off in a healthy way, not to lose the most weight in the shortest amount of time.

2. Now divide the calories from your Calorie Ceiling into separate meals and possibly a snack or two. This meal plan should fit with your personal schedule and medications. It should also work to eliminate your bad habits. It may also change from day to day, depending on what you have to do. Most of us lead hectic lives, and each day differs from the other and so can your diet.

Things to Consider

You should plan three meals a day because this makes for a strong foundation for healthy eating. Those three meals should be breakfast, lunch, and dinner, not lunch, dinner, and huge evening snack. Snacks were once seen as a necessary component for people with diabetes, but that is no longer true. You should only include a snack in your meal plan if you really want one or two a day, if you need a way to prevent your blood glucose from going too low because of your medication, or if you need snacks to eat enough calories over the course of a day.

When dividing your calories throughout the meals, you should consider your personal preferences and habits. Ask yourself questions about your daily life. Above all, a meal plan is a very personal program that must fit you. Don't try to fit your life and preferences into your meal plan; instead make it work with you. For example, if you haven't eaten breakfast in 20 years, it may be impossible to plan a 500-calorie breakfast every day. Instead, start with something very small, such as a banana and an English muffin with jam. That's simple. Here is a list of things to consider when designing your meal plan:

- What foods you enjoy and when you want to eat them.
- Your diabetes medication schedule.
- Timing and frequency of low blood glucose (hypoglycemia).
- How much food you like to eat at different meals and snacks.
- Your need or desire to include snacks.
- Your typical appetite throughout the day.
- Other dietary needs you may have, such as keeping your sodium and cholesterol levels low because of heart disease.
- How often you eat meals away from home, when, and what types of foods.
- Your weight history and attempts to lose weight.
- Your activity habits, such as times of day that you exercise, what you do, and for how long. If you're not exercising right now, you will be soon (see Chapter 21).
- Your life schedule, including your work hours if you work, how your weekdays are different from weekends, and other events in your schedule to consider.

You should try to configure your meals to how you eat and to the needs of your blood glucose levels. If dinner is currently the biggest meal during your day, then that should also be the biggest meal on your meal plan. If there is a long period between waking up and eating lunch, you should make sure that your breakfast is large enough to prevent low blood glucose. If you've noticed that your blood glucose dips lower after exercise, planning a snack before your normal exercise routine may be very helpful.

When you have made your meal plan, your doctor should be informed of this plan so that he or she can see if there are any potential conflicts between it and your medications and overall diabetes care. The worst thing that you could do is take your diabetes medication or insulin and then not eat, which could result in a dangerously low blood sugar. You may also want to meet with a registered dietitian to get help while building your meal plan. How to find a registered dietitian is described in Chapter 29.

Can This Really Work in the Real World?

Yes, this approach to eating seriously does work. As you get more comfortable with your meal plan, you can make adjustments naturally. You won't even notice a difference in your daily life once you've gotten it down.

The 1-2-3 Diabetes Diet requires common sense, and hopefully everyone has that. Really, I'm just pointing out that you need to think more carefully about how, what, and why you eat. For example, if you know that you will be splurging a little at dinner (a co-worker's birthday), then plan to have a smaller-than-normal breakfast and lunch. For those meals, you will simply cut back on your portion sizes. You might skip your snack that day to make room in your Calorie Ceiling for a slice of birthday cake. Your changes to that day's plan don't have to be perfect; an estimate will work. I'd hardly call this a magical calculation. It's quite easy, really.

If you do go over your Calorie Ceiling one day by 100 calories or so, it won't make a big difference in the grand scheme of things. The important thing to remember is that you have a Calorie Ceiling each day and do your best to stay below it. Also, don't think of your Calorie Ceiling as a weekly total. If you do go over by 100 calories one day, don't subtract 100 calories from the next day. Shifting calories back and forth from day to day can make your blood glucose levels hard to control. Just notice that you went over and move on. Work as hard as you can to keep right at your Calorie Ceiling every day.

NO NEED TO REINVENT THE WHEEL

It's not always necessary to build your meal plan from scratch. In fact, this can be the hardest way to do it. Instead, turn to the variety of meal planning systems that already exist. These systems are designed to help you automatically eat fewer calories while reducing the headache of planning. Following are just a few of the many options out there.

- Point systems. An example of this is the Weight Watchers system, which assigns points to different calorie levels. You may have 26 points to "spend" in a day, and each point may correspond to 60 or so calories. So, in essence, when you have a 26-point meal plan, you are really on a diet of 1,500 calories per day.
- Portion size. The American Diabetes Association has developed a system called Rate Your Plate. In this system, you give yourself a limited amount of food from each food group on your plate. It helps in portion control and assures that you're eating a healthy variety of foods. There are no refills or seconds and, therefore, your calorie intake is limited.
- Food delivery services, such as Seattle Sutton (*www.seattlesutton.com*), which pre-determine the calories in a meal, are another option. By eating only a limited amount of food, your calorie intake is also limited.
- *Month of Meals* series cookbooks. These American Diabetes Association cookbooks help you put together healthy daily menus that will fit into just about every meal plan. Each book offers 28 days of quick and tasty breakfast, lunch, and dinner selections, with tons of different possible combinations.

Rate Your Plate

The American Diabetes Association's Rate Your Plate is a great way to practice portion control if you are trying to lose weight. When you sit down for a meal, draw an imaginary line through the center of your plate. Draw a line to divide one section into two. Your plate is now divided into three sections.

- About one-fourth of your plate should be filled with grains or starchy foods such as rice, pasta, potatoes, corn, or peas.
- Another fourth should be protein—foods like meat, fish, poultry, or tofu.
- For the last half of your plate, you can fill it with nonstarchy vegetables like broccoli, carrots, cucumbers, salad, greens, tomatoes, and cauliflower.
- Then, add a glass of nonfat milk and a small roll or piece of fruit.
- You're ready to eat!

You may need to count the carbohydrates in your meal so that you can be sure your insulin and exercise are on target, but rating your plate will get you started. The only thing about Rate Your Plate is that while it will help in portion control and keeping diversity in your diet, it will not help you figure out your calorie count for a day.

Personally, I think that using pre-packaged or standardized meals (such as Jenny Craig or Nutrisystem) works, especially if you don't like to cook or know how to cook. These meals automatically restrict the amount of food you eat and most have a standardized calorie and nutritional content. The hard work is done for you, and all you have to do is pick which meal you will prepare. Many cookbooks have recipes for complete meals, with nutritional information and calorie content listed in the book. Just follow the directions and you have a complete meal with the calories already counted for you.

On the other hand, some people like more freedom in their diet. If you prefer not to have to follow exact meal plans, it will be helpful to do some of the hard work and research on your own to make sure that you have the knowledge to make healthy choices.

Chapter 16
Lead by Example: Joe's Weight-Loss Plan

Remember Joe? We introduced him a couple of chapters back and figured out how many calories he'd need to eat in a day to lose weight.

Joe's Calorie Ceiling

Joe weighs 220 pounds.

To maintain his weight:
$220 \times 11 = 2{,}420$ current calories.

To lose 1 pound a week:
$2{,}420 - 500 = 1{,}920$ calories a day.

To lose 2 pounds a week:
$2{,}420 - 1{,}000 = 1{,}420$ calories a day.

Let me tell you some more about Joe. He's 6 feet tall and 50 years old. He has type 2 diabetes and was diagnosed 10 years ago. By going to the BMI tables on pages 14–15, we can see that his current BMI is about 29.8, which puts him just on the verge of being obese. Joe works in an office about 10 miles from his house, so he drives a lot, and the idea of exercise makes him feel tired before he does anything. This information tells us that Joe is not an athlete or in particularly good shape, so we can trust his BMI value.

Joe's diabetes has been getting worse, so he's decided to make some changes. He's going to try to lose weight, which will help improve his blood glucose levels. His health care team sits down with him, and they do the math above. Joe decides that he should take the slow and steady route to weight loss and shoots for losing one pound a week, which means that he'll have to reduce his calorie intake to 1,920 calories a day.

Following the 1-2-3 Diabetes Diet, Joe puts together a meal plan based on the strategies we've discussed so far. Let's follow Joe to see how he puts this plan to work.

STEP ONE: THINKING ABOUT EATING

Before Joe can really get started, he'll need to keep a food diary. He does this for two weeks, continuing to eat the same way he has for as long as he can remember. He spends those two weeks objectively logging his meals and snacks in his food diary, writing things down immediately and then closing the notebook so he has little time to worry about what he's entered. Joe doesn't want to start judging himself as he makes his entries; he feels that the temptation to lie in his food diary will be too great.

STEP TWO: MAKING HEALTHY CHANGES

After two weeks, Joe sits down on a Saturday and looks at his food diary. He picked up a copy of the American Diabetes Association's *Guide to Healthy Restaurant Eating* and the *Diabetes Carbohydrate and Fat Gram Guide* so he can at least estimate how many calories he's been eating per day. He knows that he doesn't have to be perfect with the numbers of calories, but he should at least be close. He spends the afternoon tallying up his meals and adds up his daily totals for the past two weeks. He finds that he's been eating about 2,800 calories a day and realizes that if he wants to reach his goal, he'll have to take about 900 calories out of his daily eating. Joe decides not to dwell on this, finishes up his day, and decides on Sunday to look for eating patterns and habits he can change.

On Sunday, Joe knows that his goal is to reduce his calorie intake to about 1,900 calories a day; this is his Calorie Ceiling. He's not sure if he'll be able to meet it every day because he hasn't tried yet, but it's a good enough goal for the moment. But where can he cut these calories? Looking for eating habits is the key.

Finding his eating habits took Joe longer than expected. Instead of figuring it out in an afternoon, it takes a few days. Finally, though, he's come up with a small list. Here are some common traits he's found.

- Joe eats a lot more food on Fridays and Saturdays.
- Most of his at-work meals come from fast-food restaurants.
- He has a weakness for second servings at dinner. (Joe sees that he's had multiple servings of many foods every day at dinner.)
- Most of the extra calories he eats on Fridays and Saturdays come from snacks (chips, sodas, beers, etc.) he has while watching TV with his family or friends.
- His meals have a lot more meat and carbohydrates (bread, rolls, potatoes, etc.) than vegetables and fruit. In fact, he's had only one solid serving of vegetables in the last week: carrots with a pot roast. He ate no fruit over the entire two weeks.

This list is a good start. He has identified specific examples of poor eating patterns instead of generalizing and saying he eats too much. Using these examples, he decides to choose two things to change that will add up to about 900 fewer calories per day. Remembering to set realistic goals for himself, he makes these two:

1. Over the next month (*short time frame*), I will only eat lunch at a fast-food restaurant two days a week (*realistic*). The rest of the time, I will bring a healthier lunch to work (*specific* and *easy to achieve*).
2. Over the next month (*short time frame*), on Fridays and Saturdays (*specific*), I will replace my leisure-time snacks with healthier options, such as raw carrots (without dip), pretzels, and fresh fruit (*realistic* and *easy to achieve*).

These are great goals to begin Joe's weight-loss plan. If he follows through on just these two small but achievable goals, he will reduce his weekly calorie intake and improve his nutrition. Another very accessible goal for Joe would be to cut down the number of servings he has at dinner. However, Joe really enjoys having dinner with his family and his grown children often come over for meals, so he thinks that that goal may be harder to accomplish. He feels that too many emotions are tied to this eating habit, so it'll take some work to conquer this one.

With his goals in place, Joe works up to the next step: figuring out a meal plan. Joe knows that putting together his meal plan must reflect certain goals, so he writes them down to keep them in mind. Here's what Joe's list looks like:

1. My Calorie Ceiling is 1,900 calories. (Notice how Joe rounds off his Calorie Ceiling to an easy number, so he'll have an easier time matching it.)
2. I need a healthy balance to my meals, including more fruits, vegetables, and whole grains and less meat.

3. I eat three meals a day, so my meal plan should have three meals a day.
4. My daily meals are usually at the same time.
5. My diabetes medications require an evening snack.
6. Dinner is usually my biggest meal, so it should have the highest number of calories per day.

Using these guidelines, Joe draws up the following basic meal plan:

- Breakfast: 300 calories
- Lunch: 600 calories
- Dinner: 800 calories
- Evening Snack: 200 calories
- Total calories: 1,900

To make this a little more tangible and to keep him from having to estimate calories on the go, Joe decides to put together a week's worth of meals to make sure that he follows through on his new meal plan (see pages 102–103). Joe also knows that not everything he eats comes with a food label, specifically the foods he eats at restaurants, so it may work better to make most of his meals at home and bring them to work with him. He looks at the books he bought so he can make each meal pretty close to matching his Calorie Ceiling and ensure that each meal has a good balance of nutrients. His best approach is to look at what he typically eats for these meals (all of that information is already written down in his food diary) and look for healthier options to replace them. Later, when Joe becomes more comfortable with his Calorie Ceiling and monitoring what he eats, he can eat his meals, subtract that from his total Calorie Ceiling, and adjust the rest of his meals throughout the day.

This meal plan is balanced, and it stays within Joe's Calorie Ceiling. It contains some variety and focuses on many different food groups, not just meats and carbohydrates. Making this meal plan took Joe quite a while, but that effort he spent putting it together means that he can save a lot more time over the rest of the week. Many cookbooks for people with diabetes (see the Appendix) contain meal plans set at certain Calorie Ceilings, and Joe could use those to build his weekly meal plan, making the process even easier.

Notice also that Joe's meal plan contains his goals to eat less fast food and have healthier snacks on the weekends. Goals and meal plans should work together to help you lose weight. They should not be exclusive. In fact, one should help you achieve the other. For Joe, his meal plan is built around his goals, making them easy to achieve. In addition, having his goals in his meal plan makes it easier to follow it. Make sure that your goals and meal plans work together.

For the next step, Joe begins an exercise routine. He decides to go for a 30-minute walk every day when he gets home from work.

For a month, Joe will continue to keep his food diary, weigh himself three times a week on a scale, and do his best to follow through on his goals, meal plan, and exercise routine. When that month passes, he will see if he has lost weight and if his blood glucose numbers have gotten better. If things look good, he'll stick with what he's been doing and lower his Calorie Ceiling another 200 calories. If things haven't worked so well, he'll go back to his food diary and look for more patterns. He can try a number of new solutions. He could lower his Calorie Ceiling if he's kept to his meal plan or he may raise it a little bit if he's found that he eats uncontrollably because his meal plan has left him feeling starving all of the time. He could try to increase his exercise type and duration. He may also have to look at the kinds of foods he's been eating.

Important Note

Joe is a very independent person and can be stubborn at times, so he chose what may be the most difficult way to put together his meal plan—by doing research and studying books. It doesn't have to be so difficult for you. Instead, you can use a point system such as Weight Watchers or use cookbooks that contain ready-made meal plans, some of which are listed at the end of this book. Using the hard work of others to build your meal plan can reduce the amount of time spent putting together your meal plan and result in more variety in the foods you eat.

Everyone, however, should make goals based on their eating habits. It's the only way to make lasting changes to your diet and health. Make sure that you work these goals into your food plan, just like Joe did.

Joe's Meal Plan

Breakfast (300 calories)

Sunday: 1/2 cup egg substitute (70 cal), 1 cup raw vegetables (such as tomatoes, mushrooms, or spinach) (25), 1 oz low-fat cheese (55), 1 slice 90-calorie bread (90), 1 1/4 cups watermelon cubes (60), hot tea (0). Total: 300

Monday: French toast: made with 1 slice 90-calorie whole-grain bread (90 cal), 1 egg (75), cinnamon, and 1/8 cup sugar-free maple syrup (13); 1 slice lean turkey bacon (35), 6 oz nonfat milk (68). Total: 281

Tuesday: 1 cup plain oatmeal (160 cal), no-calorie sweetener, 4-oz banana (60), 8 walnut halves (90). Total: 310

Wednesday: Breakfast sandwich: made with 1 whole toasted English muffin (160 cal), 1 oz lean ham (55), and 1/4 cup egg substitute (35); 1 small orange (60). Total: 310

Thursday: 2/3 cup Mueslix (160 cal), 6 oz fat-free yogurt (90), 6 mixed nuts (45). Total: 295

Friday: 2 reduced-fat 4-inch square waffles (160 cal), 1 1/2 tsp squeeze margarine (45), 1/2 cup unsweetened applesauce (60), 1/8 cup sugar-free maple syrup (13). Total: 278

Saturday: Milkshake: made with 1 cup nonfat milk (90 cal), 1/2 cup unsweetened or other fruit (60), ice, and no-calorie sweetener; 1 slice whole-grain toast (90), 1 tsp tub margarine (45), 1/2 Tbsp low-calorie jam (13). Total: 298

Lunch (600 calories)

Sunday: Low-fat frozen meal with less than 600 mg sodium (280 cal), 8-oz apple or 1 large pear (120), 1-oz roll (80), 1 tsp soft margarine (45), 1 cup nonstarchy mixed vegetable salad (25), 2 Tbsp reduced-calorie salad dressing (45). Total: 595

Monday: Sandwich: made with 2 slices 120-calorie whole-grain bread (240 cal), 3 oz very-lean meat such as chicken (no skin) (105), 1 cup lettuce and tomato (25) and 1 Tbsp reduced-calorie mayonnaise (45); 1 small piece of fruit (such as a kiwi) (60), 3/4 oz pretzels (80), 6 mixed nuts (45). Total: 600

Tuesday: Tuna salad: made with 3 oz tuna drained of water (105 cal), mixed with 1 cup chopped mixed vegetables (25), 2 Tbsp reduced-calorie mayonnaise (90), and spices of choice over 1 cup green lettuce (25); 1 1/3 oz bread sticks (160), 13-oz orange (120), 6 oz sugar-free yogurt (90). Total: 615

Wednesday: Vegetarian burrito: made with 1 8-inch flour tortilla (110 cal), 1 cup vegetarian chili with beans (205), 1 oz low-fat cheddar cheese (50), and 1/4 avocado (85); 2 cups lettuce and tomato (50), 2 Tbsp low-fat salad dressing (80), 1 4-oz peach (60). Total: 640

Thursday: Loaded baked potato: made with a 9-oz baked potato (240 cal), 2 oz low-fat cheddar cheese (120), and 1 cup cooked broccoli (50); 6 oz diet yogurt (90), 4 ginger snaps (106). Total: 606

Friday: 2/3 cup homemade green pea soup (194 cal), 1 oz whole-wheat crackers (125), 2 oz low-fat cheese (110), 6 oz of 100-calorie yogurt (100), 1 cup cantaloupe (60). Total: 589

Saturday: Peanut butter and banana sandwich: made with 2 slices 120-calorie bread (240), 2 Tbsp regular peanut butter (200), and a 4-inch banana (80); 8 oz nonfat milk (90). Total: 610

Dinner (800 calories)

Sunday	Monday	Tuesday	Wednesday	Thursday	Friday	Saturday
4 oz baked or grilled salmon (220 cal), 6 oz baked sweet or white potato (160), 2 Tbsp reduced-fat margarine (90), 1 small roll (80), 1/2 large corn on the cob (80), 1 cup cooked asparagus (50), 1 sliced tomato (25), 8 oz nonfat milk (90). Total: 795	Spaghetti with sauce: made with 1 cup cooked pasta (240 cal) 1 cup spaghetti sauce in jar (140), and 2 oz cooked ground turkey (110) mixed in sauce; 2 cups mixed nonstarchy vegetable salad (50), 4 Tbsp reduced-calorie salad dressing (90), 1 oz dinner roll (80) dipped in 1 tsp olive oil (45), 1 cup steamed nonstarchy vegetables (50). Total: 805	4 oz barbeque dark-meat chicken (220 cal), 2 oz barbeque sauce (70), 6 oz macaroni salad (170), 1 cup cooked green beans (50), 6 almonds (45), 2-oz dinner roll (160), 1 tsp margarine (45), 1/4 cup orange juice mixed with no-calorie lemon-lime soda (30). Total: 790	Shepherd's pie: made with 3 oz lean chopped beef (165 cal), 1/2 cup gravy (50), 1 cup mashed potatoes (160), 1/2 cup peas (80), and 1 oz reduced-calorie cheddar cheese (55); 1-oz dinner roll (80), 2 tsp margarine (90), 1/2 cup cooked nonstarchy vegetables (25), 1 cup nonfat milk (90). Total: 795	4 oz porterhouse steak (220 cal), 6-oz baked sweet potato (160), 1 tsp margarine (45), 1/2 cup unsweetened applesauce (60), 1 cup cooked spinach (50), 1 slice rye bread (120), 1 tsp margarine (45), low-calorie ice cream (100). Total: 800	Breaded catfish: made with 4 oz oven-fried catfish (220 cal), 1 1/2 Tbsp cornmeal (40), and 2 tsp canola oil (90); 1/3 cup rice mixed with 1/2 cup beans (195), 1 cup Brussels sprouts (50), 1-oz brownie (125), 1 cup nonfat milk (90). Total: 810	4-oz steamed shrimp (140 cal), 2/3 cup rice (160), 1 tsp margarine (45), 13-oz orange (120), 1-oz dinner roll (80), 1 cup cooked green vegetables (50), 2 oz or 2-inch square frosted cake (205). Total: 800

Snack (200 calories)

Sunday	Monday	Tuesday	Wednesday	Thursday	Friday	Saturday
Low-fat ice-cream sandwich (140 calories, plus 2 grams fat, 1 gram saturated fat, 28 grams carbohydrate, 3 grams protein), 4 pecan halves (45). Total: 185	Half sandwich: made with 1 slice 90-calorie, whole-wheat bread (90 cal), 1/2 Tbsp peanut butter (45), and 1 Tbsp low-calorie jam (18); 4 oz nonfat milk (45). Total: 198	3 cups plain popcorn (80 cal), 1 Tbsp cheese-flavored Molly McButter (5), 10 peanuts (45), 2 Tbsp raisins (60). Total: 190	8-oz apple (120 cal), 1 Tbsp peanut butter (90). Total: 210	1/2 cup low-fat cottage cheese (70 cal), 1 cup mixed berries (such as blueberries and raspberries) (120). Total: 190	1/2 cup nonfat frozen yogurt (100 cal), 4 ginger snaps (106). Total: 206	1 cup sugar-free rice pudding (160 cal), 16 dried pistachios (40). Total: 200

Total calories

Sunday	Monday	Tuesday	Wednesday	Thursday	Friday	Saturday
1,875	1,884	1,905	1,955	1,891	1,883	1,908

Chapter 17

Smart Shopping:
How to Navigate
Your Grocery Store
and Read Food Labels

As you begin putting together your meal plans based on your Calorie Ceiling, you're going to find that eating out is one of the quickest ways to bust your calorie budget. Buying groceries and cooking at home gives you much more freedom and control over your food choices, and you'll find you can often eat more food but less calories.

Buying groceries and cooking at home are not foolproof, however. There are some common pitfalls, especially if you're used to the "old way" of shopping—that is, buying the most food at the biggest bargain. I'll give you a brief rundown on how to approach healthier habits while grocery shopping and some tips on reading food labels. Once you get used to healthy shopping, these simple activities can make creating and following a healthy meal plan easy.

SHAPING UP YOUR SHOPPING

How many times have you walked into the grocery store knowing exactly what you need, but when you're walking out to your car, you realize that you've spent more money than you wanted, bought much more food than you were intending, and even forgot to buy the things you really needed? This is not uncommon. The key tactic for the future and for following a healthy lifestyle is to take a more cautious approach to grocery shopping. Here are some tips.

- Make a shopping list and stick to it. By having a shopping list, you will be able to go directly to the items you need and buy those. You'll save money and time, and avoid buying those delicious-looking impulse items that are often belly busters.

- Don't go to the grocery store when you're hungry. You'll buy a lot more food than you planned, and you're more likely to buy junk food and unhealthy snacks if you go grocery shopping on an empty stomach.

- Do not retrace your footsteps around the grocery store. Get everything you need in each section and move to the next one. Retracing your footsteps only gives you more incentive to buy things that you don't need.

- Do not walk every aisle. If you know you do not need items in a particular aisle, don't go there. Move on to the next one, especially if they are aisles with foods that you are better off leaving behind.

- The healthiest foods in grocery stores are normally located around the edges. Fruits and vegetables will be on one wall, meats and poultry along another wall, and dairy foods against yet another wall. When you begin shopping, go around the edges first. If you fill your basket or cart with healthy items, you won't have as much space for unhealthy foods.

- When choosing specific products, look at the food labels. Compare the nutrients in one package with those in another. Choosing a low-fat mayonnaise is better than picking up the regular mayonnaise. In addition, reading food labels will allow you to make sure that what you're buying fits into your meal plan.

FOOD LABELS

I mentioned in Chapter 11 that the Nutrition Facts labels are a great way to learn the calorie content of most of the groceries we buy. Unfortunately, most of us don't pay too much attention to the labels that are on our food packages. Changing this attitude is the first and easiest step to weight loss. Once you start looking closely at the Nutrition Facts label, you begin to learn a lot about what you're putting into your body. So pay attention to the labels when you go shopping and take some time to open up your cupboard and examine the food you've got in there. You'll often find a lot of surprises.

Let's take another look at the food label from earlier in the book in more detail. If you're going to create your healthy meal plan and meet your Calorie Ceiling for the day, you are going to need to understand food labels. You should pay attention to the following parts of food labels.

1. **Serving size.** Nutrition information is given on food labels according to serving size, which is the portion size the manufacturer has indicated is standard for the product. Food manufacturers are required to list the serving size by easy-to-understand household units, for example, 1 cup, 2 tablespoons, one package, etc. Unfortunately, what is listed as the serving size on the package may not represent the amount you usually eat. In fact, many of the serving sizes listed on products are notoriously small. If possible, try to follow the suggested serving size on the food label and remember that the nutrition information represents just one serving. Therefore, if you have more than one serving of that food, you must multiply the content by the number of servings you eat. Thus, if a food has 380 calories for one serving, but you have two, you're actually eating 760 calories (380 calories × 2 servings = 760 calories).

Nutrition Facts		
Serving Size 1 cup (228g)		
Servings Per Container 2		
Amount Per Serving		
Calories 260	Calories from Fat 120	
		% Daily Value*
Total Fat 13g		**20%**
Saturated Fat 5g		**25%**
Trans Fat 2g		
Cholesterol 30mg		**10%**
Sodium 660mg		**28%**
Total Carbohydrate 31g		**10%**
Dietary Fiber 0g		**0%**
Sugars 5g		
Protein 5g		
Vitamin A 4%	•	Vitamin C 2%
Calcium 15%	•	Iron 4%

* Percent Daily Values are based on a 2,000 calorie diet. Your Daily Values may be higher or lower depending on your calorie needs.

	Calories:	2,000	2,500
Total Fat	Less than	65g	80g
Sat Fat	Less than	20g	25g
Cholesterol	Less than	300mg	300mg
Sodium	Less than	2,400mg	2,400mg
Total Carbohydrate		300g	375mg
Dietary Fiber		25g	30g
Calories per gram:			
Fat 9	•	Carbohydrate 4 •	Protein 4

2. **Calories.** This number is relatively straightforward but is important to use when considering your Calorie Ceiling for the day. Just remember that if you eat twice the listed serving size of the product, you need to double the calories listed on the package. By choosing foods with low calorie numbers, you will be able to eat larger portions of food and still stay under your Calorie Ceiling. Also pay attention to the number of Calories from Fat, which is also a good sign of how much fat is contained in a food item.

Percent (%) Daily Value

For a specific nutrient, the Percent (%) Daily Value indicates one serving's share of the total amount recommended for a day. The percentage is based on a 2,000-calorie diet. If you need more or fewer calories, then your Daily Values would be different. The Percent (%) Daily Value is a useful tool to check whether a food is high or low in a certain nutrient such as fat or fiber. A product is:

• a good source of a particular nutrient if one serving provides 10–19% of the Daily Value

• high in a nutrient if it contains 20% or more of the Daily Value

• low in that nutrient if the Daily Value is 5% or less

3. **Fat.** Although some types of fats, such as monounsaturated and polyunsaturated, are healthy, it is still important to pay attention to the overall number of calories that you consume to maintain a healthy weight. Because you are trying to lose weight, you'll want to limit the amount of fat you eat. That's where the food label comes in handy. The amount of fat per serving of a product is usually listed on the label in grams. Food labels also have a percentage amount that shows how much the fat in this food contributes to your daily total of fat. This is the Percent (%) Daily Value of fat. For example, if you eat a food that provides 40% of the recommended Daily Value of fat per day, then you should try to make sure that the rest of the foods you eat in the day add up to 60% (100% – 40% = 60%) of the recommended Daily Value. Most food labels will also show the amount of saturated fat and *trans*-fat in one serving. As we have seen earlier, these are the types of fats most linked to poor health outcomes. Choosing foods with lower levels of total fat, lower levels of recommended Daily Value, and lower levels of saturated fat and *trans*-fat will produce a healthier diet.

4. **Carbohydrates.** Carbohydrate amounts in food products are listed in grams and as Percent (%) Daily Value, just like fat. The food label lists the total carbohydrate content of the food item, which includes starches, sugars, and fiber. Most products will also include the amount of each of these types of carbohydrates on the label. As we have seen, foods higher in starches and fiber are the healthiest. But remember to look at the total amount of carbohydrate, not just the sugar.

A Note about Fiber

Fiber is good stuff, but it offers an extra bonus for people with diabetes who are counting their carbohydrates to control their blood glucose. If a food has 5 grams or more fiber in a serving, you can subtract the fiber grams from the total grams of carbohydrate for a more accurate estimate of the carbohydrate content that your body will absorb.

In addition to servings, calories, fat, and carbohydrates, food labels offer other important information on the product.

Cholesterol. Most labels list the amount of cholesterol in the food. Fortunately, cholesterol has been taken out of many manufactured products, but you should still take a look at how much of it is in your food, especially in meat products. Choosing foods lower in cholesterol is the healthy choice. An easy way to reduce the amount of cholesterol in your diet is to limit your fat intake.

Sodium. Limiting the amount of sodium you eat is important, especially if you have heart disease and high blood pressure.

Ingredient list. Looking at the ingredient list can provide important information about the nutritional value of a food product. Food labels list the ingredients in descending order according to weight. If sugar or high-fructose corn syrup is listed near the beginning of the ingredient list, it usually means that the product has high amounts of refined sugars and is a poor choice. Foods with hydrogenated and partially hydrogenated oils, such as corn oil and cottonseed oil, are less healthy choices than monounsaturated oils, such as peanut, olive, and canola oil.

FOOD CLAIMS

Now that we've talked about what you'll find printed on the labels of the foods you buy, let's talk about what you'll find printed on the front of the box. Often times, especially with foods that claim to be healthy, you see buzzwords and catchphrases that sound too good to be true. Products that are advertised as having "no added sugar" simply mean that sugar is not added during production—these foods may still contain large amounts of sugars and carbohydrates; just look at the label. "No or low fat" products may have just as many calories and more carbohydrate than the standard product. Let's explore these food claims in closer detail.

The government has defined certain claims that manufacturers may use on food packaging. For example, you'll see the claim "less sodium" on some brands of chili with beans. This means the product has at least 25% less sodium than the regular version. Some of the more popular claims are listed here.

Claims for calories

Calorie free:	less than 5 calories per serving
Low calorie:	40 calories or less per serving

Claims for fat

Fat free	less than 0.5 g of fat or saturated fat per serving
Saturated fat free	less than 0.5 g of saturated fat and less than 0.5 g of *trans*-fat per serving
Low fat	3 g or less of total fat per serving
Low saturated fat	1 g or less of saturated fat per serving
Reduced fat or less fat	at least 25% less fat than the regular version

Claims for sodium

Sodium free or salt free:	less than 5 mg of sodium per serving
Very low sodium:	35 mg of sodium or less per serving
Low sodium:	140 mg of sodium or less per serving
Reduced sodium or less sodium:	at least 25% less sodium than the regular version

Claims for cholesterol

Cholesterol free:	less than 2 mg per serving
Low cholesterol:	20 mg or less per serving
Reduced cholesterol or less cholesterol:	at least 25% less cholesterol than the regular version

Claims for sugar

Sugar free:	less than 0.5 g of sugar per serving
Reduced sugar:	at least 25% less sugar per serving than the regular version

Claims for fiber

High fiber:	5 g or more of fiber per serving
Good source of fiber:	2.5 g to 4.9 g of fiber per serving

Quick Tips for Healthy Grocery Store Choices

When thinking about buying something at the grocery store, look at its food label and ask yourself these questions:

- Is the portion size realistic for you or will you need to count it as more than one serving?
- How many calories and carbohydrates are in a serving?
- How many grams of fat are in a serving? Will eating this food push you over your recommended Percent Daily Value of fat in a day?
- Do the advertising and nutrition claims on the package match the Nutrition Facts?
- Are you comfortable with this food in your house, or is it better to avoid the temptation?
- If it is a convenience, ready-to-eat food that is likely to be expensive, can you make it at home? A homemade recipe can be less expensive, be lower in calories and sodium, and have fewer additives.

Chapter 18
Six Food Myths
That Need to Be Busted

Eating healthy requires that you also have some knowledge of what makes a healthy diet. You'll often hear "common wisdom" about food and healthy eating that is just plain wrong. It's even worse if you have diabetes. There are many myths surrounding diabetes and diet that are popular but simply are not true. In this chapter, I'll lay to rest some of the more common myths you may have already heard or will hear in the future.

1. Eating a lot of fat makes you fat.

Eating too much fat does not make you fat. Eating more calories than you use or need makes you fat. That said, it is smart to limit the fat you eat. Fat has more than twice as many calories as carbohydrates or protein, so eating more fat often means eating more calories. Everyone should limit their intake of saturated fat, which can raise your bad cholesterol, and *trans*-fat, which can raise bad cholesterol and may lower good cholesterol.

2. Eating sugar gives you diabetes or, if you already have it, makes it worse.

Eating sugar does not cause diabetes. Too much sugar is not the problem. The problem is eating too much food—all types of food—especially foods high in calories. Eating too many calories can make you overweight, and being overweight can lead to type 2 diabetes. It's true that eating a piece of cake made with sugar will raise your blood glucose level, but so will eating corn on the cob, a baked potato, or lima beans. People with diabetes can and do eat

But Watch Out for Sugary Drinks

There is one thing to keep in mind about sugar, however. When sugar enters your body in liquid form, it is digested or broken down faster than sugar in solid foods, causing blood glucose spikes after you eat. So be careful when drinking regular soda, fruit juice (this includes 100% fruit juices, too), and other sweetened drinks because controlling your blood glucose levels during these spikes can be difficult. You'll be better off if you drink water, flavored water, unsweetened iced tea, and other similar drinks instead.

sugar. In your body, it becomes glucose, just like the other foods mentioned above. With sugary foods, the rule is moderation. Eat too much, and *1)* you'll send your blood glucose level up higher than you expected; *2)* you'll fill up, but without the nutrients that come with vegetables and grains; and *3)* you'll gain weight. So, don't pass up that occasional slice of birthday cake. Instead, eat a little less bread or potato over the day and replace it with the cake. Taking a brisk walk is also always helpful.

3. Fat-free foods are guilt-free foods.

Even if it says it's fat free, you still need to watch the calories and portion size. Fat-free foods still have calories, often as many as their full-fat versions, and those calories count just the same as any other calories. The same is true for sugar-free foods. You should compare the calories in a fat-free or sugar-free food to the "regular" version by looking at the nutrition labels. Right now, watching calories is your first priority.

4. Foods that claim "no sugar added" contain no sugar at all.

Foods that say they have "no sugar added" can still have sugar. This only means that no extra sugar has been added. "No sugar added" foods may naturally contain other types of sugar that may have just as many calories.

5. Eating protein helps build muscle.

Eating protein does not build muscle. Bigger muscles come from muscle-building exercise. The average American diet contains more protein than it needs to build and maintain muscle.

6. Foods need to be eaten in special combinations to be digested properly.

A healthy diet doesn't require eating a certain combination of foods at each meal. This doesn't mean, however, that your diet shouldn't be varied. Eating a wide variety of foods throughout the day is the key to a healthy diet.

Chapter 19
The Truth about Carbohydrates

The popularity of low-carb diets over the past few years has been incredible. In fact, you may have tried such a diet yourself, most likely with mixed results. While this trend is starting to fade, in its wake is a lot of confusion about carbohydrates. With all of this media hubbub, the words "carb," "carbohydrate," and "net carbs" are tossed about with such frequency that for the normal person, understanding what's being discussed becomes a puzzling mess. What is the truth about carbohydrates?

Carbohydrates are found in many foods and have a greater immediate effect on your blood glucose level than any other foods, such as protein and fat. When considering diabetes and weight loss, it is important to think of carbohydrates as occurring as three types:

1. Sugars. These are the most basic carbohydrates. Examples include sucrose (table sugar), glucose, fructose (fruit sugar), and lactose (milk sugar). Because these carbohydrates consist of only a few molecules of carbohydrate put together, they are easily broken down into glucose in the bloodstream and used for energy. Sugars break down quickly, which is why some people can experience "sugar rushes" after eating them. Even though these carbohydrates break down quickly, medical research has not shown that these carbohydrates have any different effect on your blood sugar than other carbohydrates.

2. Starches. These types of carbohydrates are composed of carbohydrates linked together. Starches are found in grains, bread, rice, pasta and cereal, some fruits, and some vegetables, such as beans and potatoes. Because of the multiple molecular bonds that make up these carbohydrates, it takes your body longer to break down starches than it does sugars. Understandably, this slower process of digesting means that they provide a steady source of energy, but their effect on your blood glucose is generally the same as that for sugars. Foods that contain starches often contain fiber as well, which is very important in a healthy diet.

3. Fiber. Fiber is a type of carbohydrate that is indigestible to humans. Fiber is found in fruits, vegetables, beans, and nuts. Because it is not absorbed into the bloodstream, fiber has no noticeable calories.

The proper place for carbohydrates in a healthy diet is disputed among many scientists. Some health care providers suggest low-carb diets while others suggest increasing certain types of carbohydrates. The confusion doesn't end there. There is even debate as to which type of carbohydrate raises blood glucose levels the fastest. In the

Q&A

Wait, I think I've heard of the glycemic index before. What is it?
The glycemic index is a meal-planning tool for diabetes that ranks foods containing carbohydrate according to their potential to raise blood glucose levels. Pure glucose, which induces the greatest blood glucose response, has a glycemic index of 100. Other foods are ranked according to how quickly they cause a change in blood sugar, in comparison to their response to pure glucose.

Generally, carbohydrate foods that break down quickly during digestion, such as most flaked breakfast cereals, have the highest glycemic index values. Those that break down slowly, such as fiber-rich cereals, release glucose gradually into the bloodstream and have lower glycemic index values. Other factors that influence the glycemic index of a food are the amount of fat it contains, the type of starch it's composed of, the physical form of the food, its fiber content, and the cooking and processing methods used during its preparation.

The glycemic index is used mainly in Europe and Australia, but recommendations in the United States suggest that basing your diet solely on the glycemic index is unwise. For example, potato chips and French fries have a lower glycemic index than a baked potato, but you should consider their fat content as well as their effect on blood glucose. Many foods containing refined sugar have a moderate glycemic index, but their empty calories still mean that they shouldn't become a major part of your diet. The complexity of the glycemic index makes it a challenge to put it into practice.

past, because sugars are easier to break down than starches, many scientists believed that sugars raised blood glucose levels quickest. More recently, however, studies have indicated that certain types of starches (such as those found in breads or potatoes) will cause a quicker rise in blood glucose than sugars. This eventually led to a rating system you may have heard of before, called the glycemic index. This index generally indicates which foods raise blood sugar the fastest. With all of this confusing and contradictory science concerning carbohydrates, it is no wonder people become confused when figuring out how many carbohydrates to put in their diet.

QUICK THOUGHTS ON CARBOHYDRATE

Here are some simple guidelines to keep in mind while thinking about carbohydrates, diabetes, and your diet.

1. Carbohydrates by themselves are not bad. In fact, they are a necessary part of any person's healthy diet. In our American diet, carbohydrates aren't the whole problem; it's usually the stuff added to the carbohydrates that pose the problem. For example, it is the butter, cream, and fat added to carbohydrates that greatly increase the calories. So while a small baked potato has about 300 calories, adding butter, sour cream, and bacon bits will make the whole thing add up to 500 or 600 calories. We need to learn to drop these extra calories from what would otherwise be healthy carbohydrates. Just keep in mind that with diabetes, you must pay attention to your carbohydrate intake because of its effect on your blood glucose levels.

2. Americans love fried foods. The list goes on forever: French fries, hush puppies, hash browns, mozzarella sticks, fried bananas, fried ice cream, fried candy bars, fish sticks, and so on. Although you may start out with a wholesome carbohydrate like a potato, by the time you slice it and fry it into French fries, you have greatly increased its number of calories and its amount of fat and cholesterol.

3. Portion sizes of carbohydrates are often way too large. Some of this comes from portion sizes that are too big in general, and some comes from the "if it's fat-free, I can eat as much as I want" myth we discussed last chapter. Fat-free foods are often rich in carbohydrates, which still contain calories. Again, a few slices of a potato, cooked in a healthy way with little added fat, are a good addition to your diet. Eating half of a bag of potato chips in a sitting is not.

4. Refined and processed carbohydrates are usually not healthy.

Keywords: Empty Calories

Sometimes people tell me that they are eating well below their Calorie Ceiling, yet they continue to gain weight and their blood glucose levels worsen. To get to the bottom of the problem, we'll look at their food diaries and find a bunch of snacks that haven't been counted in their daily totals. When I ask them why, they'll say, "Oh, those were empty calories, so those don't count." This is nutrition confusion at its most dangerous.

Many people have heard the term "empty calories" applied to sodas, chips, and other junk foods. Unfortunately, they misunderstand what this means. Instead of meaning "no calories," the term "empty calories" means that the foods still have calories—often a lot of calories—just relatively little to no nutritional value. When you eat a food filled with empty calories, you're adding these calories to your daily intake, but you're not getting any vitamins or any healthy amounts of vital nutrients in return. This is why they're "empty." When you have diabetes and you need to lose weight, one of the most important actions you can take is to reduce the number of foods you eat with empty calories.

Store-bought baked goods and frozen meals are usually laden with calories. So are processed foods such as snack chips, cookies, and crackers. In addition, these foods are often lacking in other nutritional value. These are what we call "empty calories." Again, we should not entirely blame the carbohydrates found in these items, but we need to also look at the fat, calorie, and nutritional value of these foods. This is why you should look at food labels whenever possible.

5. Fiber is good. The health benefits of a high-fiber diet are well known. Increased dietary fiber can lower bad cholesterol levels and has been connected to lower levels of intestinal disorders and lower frequencies of certain types of cancer.

CARBOHYDRATES AND THE 1-2-3 DIABETES DIET

I've developed the 1-2-3 Diabetes Diet to be your starting point on the road to healthy eating and weight loss. To make this process simpler, I've decided to focus more on counting calories than counting carbohydrates. But people with diabetes should not take carbohydrates lightly—too much carbohydrate will make your blood glucose levels soar sky high. The key to incorporating carbohydrates into your diet is in maximizing the right type of carbohydrate. Here are some suggestions for a healthy carbohydrate intake.

1. Try to choose carbohydrates that are whole-grain and contain fiber. Whole-wheat and whole-grain breads, pastas, rice, and bagels contain more fiber than the processed (or refined) white carbohydrates in white bread, pastries, and junk foods.

2. Choose carbohydrates that are fresh. Usually, the more a food is processed, the more fat and calories it probably contains and the

less added nutrition you will get in your diet. Fresh fruits and vegetables are usually the best carbohydrate choices.

3. Do not cover your carbohydrates with sauces that are high in fat; this includes butter and cream.

4. Cut down on fried food in your diet. If you want to remove some type of carbohydrate from your diet, choose to eliminate French fries and breaded foods first.

5. Limit portion sizes. As always, remember to limit the amount of whatever carbohydrate you are eating to fit this into your Calorie Ceiling.

Later on, when you have become comfortable with meeting your Calorie Ceiling, losing weight, and following a regular exercise routine, you can start counting your carbohydrates to improve your blood glucose control. That, however, is a more advanced technique, but by counting calories, you will learn the tools that are necessary to succeed in counting carbohydrates. Counting carbohydrates is covered in Chapter 28.

Chapter 20

Some Foods to Consider: Calorie Bargains and Budget Busters

When it comes to losing weight and taking care of your diabetes, there really aren't any good guys or bad guys. You can eat many of the same foods you ate before as long as you focus on portion size and balance your eating with healthy options. On the other hand, avoiding some foods when you start out will be easier than tempting fate altogether. Here, I'll describe four foods that make it easy to stay under your Calorie Ceiling and seven foods you should try to avoid when you're starting out.

FOODS THAT DON'T COUNT

We are lucky to have some foods that have such a minimal number of calories that they do not need to be counted in your daily Calorie Ceilings. These foods can be used to further balance your diet, stretch your Calorie Ceiling, and serve as emergency snacks when the dreaded hunger hits.

1. **Water:** Water is the perfect food. Water has no calories and is essential for good health. While most humans can survive weeks without food, we all know that humans can survive only a few days without water. Water cleanses the body, provides much of our body mass, and quenches our thirst. Water can also replace high-calorie drinks at most meals, allowing you to fill up on solid foods while staying below your Calorie Ceiling. Make sure that you drink at

least four 8-ounce glasses of water a day.

2. **Sugar-free and calorie-free drinks and snacks:** In my eyes, one of the most innovative recent inventions is the artificial sweetener. These calorie-free sugar substitutes allow us to eat sugary-tasting products without the calories. There are countless sugar-free and calorie-free items available—from soft drinks to lemonade to candy. I am always surprised that dieters do not use these products more. However, the health risks of consuming large quantities of these products are largely unknown, so use them in moderation, as small occasional snacks. The other danger is that some products, although sugar free, are not calorie free (they instead contain fat, protein, and carbohydrates other than sucrose). Careful label reading is the key to success here.

A Potential Downside to Artificial Sweeteners

Some recent studies focusing on artificial sweeteners and their effects on weight loss have produced some surprising results. Mainly, that people who drink or eat a lot of artificial sweeteners sometimes actually gain more weight than those who don't. While the reasons for this are still unclear, one possibility is that artificial sweeteners stimulate hunger and cause people to overeat. This is no reason to cut out artificial sweeteners completely—they still allow us to enjoy some foods we wouldn't get to enjoy otherwise. However, if you find you're absolutely starving after a diet soda, try drinking more water or tea instead.

---

3. **Small quantities of raw vegetables.** Not only does a small helping of raw carrots or celery provide a healthy snack, they also contain almost no calories at all. Just remember to stay away from dips and sauces. This is not to say that you shouldn't eat raw vegetables in larger quantities, just that if you have a few for a snack, you're not taking in too many calories.

4. **Herbs and spices.** No one said eating healthy has to be dull. When low-calorie, low-fat foods start to get boring, spice it up a little. Herbs and spices add a whole new level of taste to your foods and, best of all, have no effect on your diabetes control. Some popular spice mixes, such as garlic salt, do contain sodium, so you should be careful with these.

The Spice of Life

Here is a brief list of possible spices and foods they complement well.

- *Garlic:* beef, poultry, potatoes, pasta
- *Rosemary:* lamb, poultry, potatoes
- *Dill weed:* seafood, salads, fish, shellfish, poultry
- *Tarragon:* poultry, rice, beef, lamb, pork
- *Oregano:* lamb, pasta, chili, poultry
- *Ginger:* chicken, pork, polenta, some desserts
- *Paprika:* potatoes, pasta, beef, poultry
- *Mint:* chicken, lamb, pork, pasta, fruit

This list is hardly complete. There are tons of spices out there and just as many flavorful combinations, so feel free to experiment while cooking. Dried herbs and spices, like the ones you normally see on grocery store shelves, store for a long time and are much stronger than fresh ones, so be prepared to try many combinations.

FOODS TO AVOID

Some foods have so many calories, are laden with so much fat, or are so filled with empty calories that most of us should just avoid them completely when trying to follow a healthy diet. At least try to cut down on how much of these foods you eat. Unfortunately, many of these items also taste great because of the very fat and empty calories that make them bad for you. To make matters worse, these foods are often the most heavily advertised items you'll see.

1. French fries. Americans love their French fries. In many restaurants it is difficult to find a healthy side dish to substitute for French fries without spending extra money. In addition, the portion size of French fries has grown ridiculously in the past few decades. French fries offer little nutritional value, and they pack a hefty load of calories and *trans*-fats. Do yourself a favor and drop the French fry addiction.

2. Fast-food breakfast sandwiches and burgers. These items are among the unhealthiest items available in America. The fat and calories contained in one breakfast sandwich or specialty hamburger often reaches 50–75% of your allotted fat and calories for the whole day. Do yourself a second favor and get rid of the fast-food addiction altogether.

3. "Americanized" Italian food. This group includes pizza, cream sauces (Alfredo sauce, for example), and garlic bread. Italian food can be healthy. In fact, Mediterranean cuisine made with fresh vegetables, olive oil, and small portions of meat is a great, healthy diet option. Unfortunately, Americans have turned Italian food into fat-laden meals of huge portion sizes, particularly at "family-style" restaurants, which often serve enough food for three people on one plate. Authentic Italian cuisine rarely features fried mozzarella sticks or cheese-stuffed pizzas.

4. Alcoholic beverages. Large quantities of alcoholic beverages contain many empty calories, which is why we call that belly a "beer gut." Most alcoholic beverages, like beer, also contain carbohydrates, which will affect your blood glucose level. When it comes to balancing diabetes and drinking alcohol, you must be moderate in your habits and plan carefully. On the other hand, many recent studies have shown that *moderate alcohol consumption* can have beneficial health effects. What does this mean? Moderate drinking is defined as two drinks a day for men and one drink a day for women. A drink is defined as a 5-ounce glass of wine, a 12-ounce light beer, or 1 1/2 ounces of 80-proof distilled spirits. Also, if you are going to drink, make sure that it won't interfere with your medications.

5. Ice cream and snack foods. For many people, the nutritional value of their daily meals is reasonable. Unfortunately, some people fill the hours between these more-or-less nutritious meals with large quantities of snack foods, usually during the evening. Snacking all night in front of the TV is an eating habit you will have to break if you are going to follow a healthy meal plan. Remember, we call it junk food for a reason.

6. Fried ethnic or regional foods. Every culture seems to have at least one treasured high-fat, fried food item. Whether it is a deep-fried burrito (*chimichanga*), an egg roll, hush puppies, or that perfect Southern-style fried chicken, you need to avoid these items as much as possible until you are able to manage your meal plan, Calorie Ceiling, and blood glucose levels effectively. As always, if the food comes fried, covered in sauce, or in a huge portion, it will not fit into your healthy meal plan. Almost every restaurant has healthy options; just look.

7. Real mayonnaise and sauces. Sauces and condiments such as mayonnaise often make a meal. Other tasty toppings often double as dipping sauces—bleu cheese and ranch dressings, for example. Unfortunately, all of these can add more calories and fat to your diet than the food they are covering. There are healthy sauces, made without fat and oil, and you will want to switch to those. If you absolutely can't live without the mayonnaise, salad dressing, or creamy sauce, try having it put on the side of the dish. By putting the sauces on the side, you will often have less of it than normal and can control how much of it you are actually eating.

A Word to the Wise

Keep in mind that for some of us, simply cutting the things we like out of our diet (or any part of our lives, for that matter) may actually make us crave it more, setting us up for dangerous binge eating. Don't feel bad about having these cravings; it's perfectly human to feel this way. For example, let's say you absolutely love French fries and used to eat them with two meals a day. You try to completely cut them out of your diet and you go three days without any. The next thing you know, you get a monster craving for French fries and go out and eat two full orders of fries in one sitting. Now you've "fallen off the wagon" and can't stop ordering French fries.

Does this scenario sound familiar? If you've ever dieted before, it probably does. The point of the 1-2-3 Diabetes Diet is to keep situations like this from happening in the first place. If cutting this food out your diet is too difficult, your first step should be to cut down on how much you eat of it, not cut it out completely. Try to eat French fries only twice a week. If you do "fall off the wagon," don't let this discourage you. Just get right back on. You need to cut down on unhealthy foods, but you need to approach it in a practical way.

Everyone operates differently when it comes to their eating habits, so find the approach that works for you. After all, some people may find it easier to quit French fries "cold turkey," rather than gradually cutting down. Making it not an option at all helps these individuals move on and consider other food choices. It's all about finding a balance that works for you.

Chapter 21
Exercise

You knew it was coming, and there's no point in trying to avoid it. If you want to lose weight and stay healthy, you will absolutely need to exercise at least three days a week. A lot of magic pills and fad diets propose that you can burn away fat while sitting in your chair. They tell you that you won't have to lift a finger to lose excess weight because the magic solution will invisibly do all of that dirty work for you. This is nonsense. Even if you could burn off pounds while sitting in front of the TV, think of all of the other health benefits you'd be missing without any physical activity. Exercise does more than make you lose weight; it strengthens your lungs, heart, and muscles. You can't get that from sitting still.

Regular exercise provides countless benefits to everyone, but people with diabetes should make a standard exercise routine a key component of their lifestyles. Exercise, however, requires hard work, sweat, and time, and most people see this as enough of a bother to never exercise. I will be the first to admit that regular exercise can be a pain. We all know that it is much easier to sit in front of the TV than work out on the treadmill. If you need some motivating thoughts on why you should exercise, go back to Chapter 9 and remember that we are talking about your health and your life here. You can lose weight by reducing your calorie intake, but nothing makes a body trim like exercise. Trust me; you'll even start to feel a lot better about yourself after you begin exercising regularly.

THE BASICS OF EXERCISE

There are three types of exercise: aerobic exercise, strength training, and flexibility training. All of these have great benefits for your health and you should incorporate some element from each into your exercise routine.

Aerobic Exercise

Aerobic exercise works out the heart, lungs, arms, and legs. It increases your heart rate, works your muscles, raises your breathing rate, and burns calories. This is the best type of exercise for weight loss. To get the best results from aerobic exercise, you must exert yourself at a steady level for an extended period of time. Examples of aerobic exercise include walking, running, swimming, and biking. Aerobic sports involve constant motion and include activities such as tennis, jumping rope, and basketball.

Remember, the more strenuous the activity and the longer you do it, the more benefits you get. Aerobic exercise builds endurance and increases your energy. Some people find that it helps them sleep better, reduces stress, balances emotions, and generally improves feelings of well-being. But that's not all. Aerobic exercise can make your insulin work more efficiently, in addition to burning fat and calories. Here is a list of common aerobic activities and the amount of calories burned in a 30-minute session.

Calories Burned during Aerobic Exercise

These calculations are based on a 5'10" man weighing 154 pounds. If you weigh more, you will burn more calories. On the other hand, if you weigh less, you'll burn fewer calories.

Type of Exercise	Calories Burned in 30 Minutes
Dancing	165
Walking (3 1/2 miles per hour)	140
Swimming	255
Running/jogging (5 miles per hour)	295
Golf (walking, not riding)	165

Strength Training

This type of exercise involves lifting weights or working out on weight machines. It also includes other activities, such as using medicine balls, using exercise bands (big rubber bands), and doing calisthenics (for example, push-ups, pull-ups, and sit-ups). Strength training builds muscles and burns calories, but at a slower pace than aerobic exercise. An important benefit to strength training is that as you build more muscle, you will burn more calories, even while at rest. Scientific research has also shown that increasing your muscle mass can reduce insulin resistance and lower blood glucose levels.

Keep in mind that strength training, like all exercise, can lead to injuries. Be sure not to overexert yourself while lifting weights, and check with your doctor before beginning a rigorous program. Stretch before and after lifting weights. Keep breathing when you lift weights. Choose a range of exercises that will work out several different groups of muscles. Be sure to allow 48 hours between these sessions, so your muscles can recover and you can avoid injury.

Flexibility Exercises

Flexibility exercises, or stretching, are a vital part of a healthy exercise routine. Stretching ensures that your joints stay flexible and reduces your chance of injuring yourself when doing other exercises. Stretching should be an everyday activity and a part of every exercise workout. You'll find that the more you stretch, the more flexible you will become over time.

Some forms of exercise are based almost exclusively on flexibility, and include activities such as yoga, martial arts, and Pilates. These activities burn calories, but at a lower rate than aerobic exercise. For these dedicated flexibility exercises, you'll also have to find an instructor to properly learn the exercises. Be sure to check with your health care provider to see if there are any problems for a person with your health issues when following these exercises. Also find out if the exercise instructor is familiar with diabetes. On a final note, yoga and Pilates programs seem to relax many people, which must have some health benefit.

Guidelines for Stretching
- Stretch slowly and smoothly.
- Remember to breathe.
- Don't bounce.
- Relax and let go of any tension you feel.
- Go only as far as you can without pain.
- Try to hold for 15–20 seconds.

How Long and How Often?

If you haven't exercised regularly (or at all) for a long time, you should ease into a regular exercise routine. This means starting slowly. As a rule, aim for exercising 30 minutes a day for five days a week. Ideally, 60 minutes a day is the best way to improve your health, but doing so requires so much time in a person's already-busy schedule that most of us cannot achieve that goal. A good goal will be to exercise vigorously for at least 30 minutes straight, but when you start out just try to make your total activity over the day add up to 30 minutes. Taking three 10-minute brisk walks over the course of a day will be a helpful introduction. Make it a point to not overexert yourself while exercising. Doing so can prove dangerous.

Exercising for less than 15 minutes a day is not likely to improve your health. Gradually build up to 20 to 60 minutes of continuous aerobic exercise three to five times a week. This time does not count the time you use for warm ups and cool downs. Warm up for about 5 to 10 minutes prior to exercising, doing stretches and light work to increase your heart rate. Cool-down periods are just as important. You should gently stretch or walk for about 5 to 10 minutes after you are finished exercising.

Remember to mix up your exercises over a week. Do some weight lifting two or three days a week. Walk around the neighborhood for another two or three days a week and gradually increase your level of aerobic exercise. Start and finish each session with some stretching.

There's also something called *incidental exercise*, which is when you perform a physical activity outside of your normal daily exercise routine, but as a common lifestyle activity. This is often a great source of exercise when it becomes habit. After all, the more you move around, the more energy you'll have. Increasing your daily activity means that you burn even more calories, achieving greater weight loss. Here are some handy examples.

- Walk instead of drive whenever possible. This also includes taking a parking spot farther away from your destination than right next to the front door.

- Take the stairs instead of the elevator.

- Do some housecleaning or garden work every day. Scrubbing bathtubs can build up a sweat.

- Put away the TV remote control. Get up and walk to the TV to change channels. Better yet, turn the set off and do something else that is physical.

- Walk around while talking on the phone.

Signs That You Are Exercising Too Hard

- You can't talk while exercising.
- Your heartbeat (pulse) feels very fast.
- You consider your level of exertion as hard or very hard.

If any of the above applies to your exercise routine, you should stop immediately and reconsider what you are doing for physical activity. Exercise should not equal torture. It should require effort, but not become an impossible task. Tone down your routine and start slower.

TIPS ON GETTING STARTED

Here are some important things you should keep in mind when starting an exercise routine.

- Plan a safe exercise routine. Different exercises work out different parts of the body, and certain health conditions can affect how our bodies respond to specific exercises. For example, people with heart problems should be careful when doing aerobic exercises. Your health care provider will be able to tell you if an exercise routine will affect your heart, blood vessels, eyes, kidneys, feet, and nervous system in any negative ways.

- Have a plan. Think about what activities are realistic for you and choose the ones you think you can do. Start slowly. Your activity should be somewhat challenging but not overly difficult. Write down exactly what you'll do, where and when you'll do it, how often, and for how long. Allow yourself to get into a routine. Be flexible, and don't get discouraged. For example, get off the bus one stop earlier. Don't be too hard on yourself if you can't do this. If it's raining, you may not want to walk outside, so you can choose a different activity. It's more important to reach your long-term goal than to follow the plan exactly from day to day.

- Reward yourself. A lot of the benefits of exercise come slowly, so keep yourself motivated by planning rewards. For example, if you exercise five days a week, treat yourself to that movie you've wanted to see for so long. Or maybe you've just increased your exercise time to 45 minutes a day; buy yourself those shoes you've been staring at for weeks. Just make sure that your rewards don't undo all of your hard work. Eating a huge fast-food meal, for example, will only set you back. Your rewards should also be short term. You shouldn't reward yourself with two weeks of no exercise, for example. One day might be fine, but you don't want to discourage yourself from following through on your healthy lifestyle changes.

- Wear a medical identification bracelet. These bracelets, necklaces, or tags contain information about your health status and let anyone know that you have diabetes if anything happens. These are vital if you were to fall unconscious or if no one who knows you is around.

- Track your progress. You may find it motivating to write down what physical activity you've done each day. For example, you can make a note of what you did and how long you did it. Some people enjoy using a step counter, also called a pedometer, to see how far they've walked. Ask you health care provider where to get one.

OVERCOMING BARRIERS

As people, we don't want to exercise. It just requires too much of us. If you're like me, one of the best things about graduating high school was that I wouldn't be forced to exercise in gym class ever again in my life. That's not a very positive attitude, though. Exercise provides so many health benefits that it's hard to justify not exercising. Plus, our bodies are made to move, not sit around all night watching TV. Here are some common reasons (or barriers) why people say they can't or won't exercise and some tactics to help you overcome them.

I don't have time to exercise for 30 minutes a day.
Do as much as you can. Every step counts. If you're just starting out, start with 10 minutes a day and add more little by little. Work up to 10 minutes at a time, three times a day. Like everything else that is a priority in your life, you will need to dedicate time in your day for exercise.

I'm too tired after work.
Plan to do something active before work or during the day.

I don't have the right clothes.
Wear anything that's comfortable as long as you have shoes that fit well and socks that don't irritate your skin.

I'm too shy to exercise in a group.
Choose an activity you can do on your own, such as following along with an aerobics class on TV, using an exercise video, or going for a walk.

I don't want to have sore muscles.

Exercise shouldn't hurt if you go slowly at first. Choose something you can do without getting sore. Learn how to warm up and stretch before you do something active and how to cool down afterward.

I'm afraid I'll get low blood glucose.

If you're taking a medication that could cause low blood glucose, talk to your health care provider about ways to exercise safely.

Walking hurts my knees.

Try chair exercises, armchair aerobics videos, water aerobics, or swimming.

It's too hot outside.

If it's too hot, too cold, or too humid, walk inside a shopping center.

It's not safe to walk in my neighborhood.

Find an indoor activity, such as an exercise class at a community center, or location, such as a shopping center.

I'm afraid I'll make my condition worse.

Get a checkup before planning your fitness routine. Learn what's safe for you to do.

I can't afford to join a fitness center or buy equipment.

Do something that doesn't require fancy equipment, such as walking, jumping rope, or using cans of food for weights.

Exercise is boring.

They say variety is the spice of life. Try different activities on different days until you find something that you enjoy doing.

DIABETES AND EXERCISE

Beginning to exercise when you haven't been active for a long time is always going to be a difficult process. But when you have diabetes to top it off, there are a lot of things you need to consider. Here are some things you should know about combining an exercise routine with proper diabetes care.

Blood Glucose and Physical Activity

Exercise can affect a person's blood glucose level in random ways. No person, it seems, has the exact same blood glucose reaction to exercise. Generally, exercise makes blood glucose levels go down. Some medications lower blood glucose levels, so combining these with exercise can be potentially dangerous. However, if your blood glucose level is high before you start exercising, the physical activity can send your blood glucose levels even higher. The trick to exercising with diabetes is to find out how you personally react to physical activity. This means you should check your blood glucose frequently before and after exercise. Here are four tips for determining your blood glucose reaction to exercise.

1. *Check your blood glucose twice before exercise, once at 30 minutes before and again just before exercising.* If you do this, you can determine whether your blood glucose is rising or falling. Make sure that your blood glucose is stable before beginning exercise.

2. *Be ready to check your blood glucose during exercise.* You may want to keep an eye on your blood glucose levels during exercise, especially when you begin a new routine, when you feel like your blood glucose is going low, and when you exercise for long periods (an hour or more). Don't ignore the results. If you see that your blood glucose is falling, then treat it with a carbohydrate snack. If your blood glucose is 70 mg/dl or lower, treat it immediately.

3. *Check your blood glucose after exercise.* Your body continues to take up glucose from the blood after exercise—a process that can take hours. During this time, your glucose levels can continue to fall. Be sure to check your blood glucose often.

4. *Put yourself in a learning situation.* Like many other things we've talked about in this book, understanding your blood glucose response to exercise is a learning process. As you check your blood glucose over a span of time, look for patterns that will help you understand how your body reacts to exercise. As you begin to understand yourself better, you won't need to check your blood glucose as frequently, but can instead check it when you've noticed changes before.

Should I Eat Snacks?

Depending on how hard and how long you exercise, you may need to eat additional snacks to keep your blood glucose at an acceptable level. This is especially true for people who use insulin or medications that can cause hypoglycemia. If you do not take insulin or use these meds, a snack is usually not necessary. Generally, these snacks should contain 15 grams of carbohydrate. You may need to eat a snack before, during, or after exercise. To stay within your Calorie Ceiling, shift some food to this snack time rather than add extra food.

Suggested Snacks for Exercise

- 1 small piece of fruit
- 1 cup yogurt
- 1/2 English muffin or bagel
- 1 small muffin
- 2 Tbsp raisins
- 6–8 oz sports drink
- 4–5 snack crackers
- 1/4 cup dried fruit
- 1/2 snack bar

Snacking: When and How Much?

If you take insulin or oral medications that can lead to hypoglycemia, follow these guidelines for snacking and exercise.

If your blood glucose level is less than 100 mg/dl before exercise:
You may need to eat a snack before you begin.

If your blood glucose level is between 100 and 150 mg/dl before exercise AND you will be exercising for more than 1 hour:
You will need to eat 15 grams of carbohydrate every 30 minutes to 1 hour.

If your blood glucose level is between 100 and 250 mg/dl before exercise AND you will be exercising for less than 1 hour:
You probably will not need to eat a snack before you start.

If your blood glucose level is below 100 mg/dl during exercise:
You may need to eat a snack during exercise.

If your blood glucose level is below 100 mg/dl after exercise:
You may need to eat a snack after exercise.

What Should I Drink?

When you exercise, you sweat. When you sweat, your body loses fluid, which can result in dehydration if untreated. You should make it a point to keep yourself hydrated before, during, and after exercise. Try to drink water. It's good for you and usually the best and healthiest choice. However, if you've been exercising for a long time (an hour or more), then you may want a drink that contains carbohydrate. Be sure to choose drinks that are no more than 10% carbohydrate (read the food label), such as sports drinks and diluted fruit juices.

When Should I Exercise?

A good time to exercise is one to three hours after you finish a meal or snack. The food you have eaten will help keep your blood glucose level from falling too low. This may not be true if you are using rapid-acting insulin. If this is the case, talk with your health care provider about the appropriate time to exercise.

On the other hand, here are some guidelines on when not to exercise:

- Your blood glucose level stays over 300 mg/dl.

- Your insulin or diabetes pills are peaking.

- You have ketones in your urine.

- You have numbness, tingling, or pain in your feet or legs.

- You are short of breath.

- You are ill.

- You have a serious injury.

- You feel dizzy.

- You feel sick to your stomach.

- You have pain or tightness in your chest, neck, shoulders, or jaw.

- You have blurred vision or blind spots.

If unusual symptoms arise, report them to your health care team as soon as possible.

THE BOTTOM LINE

You've just read a lot of information on exercise, and I'm sure it all sounds like a lot of work. Some of what you've read may be discouraging. After all, if you have heart problems, I've shown you probably shouldn't be sprinting 3 miles on a treadmill. Remember this: absolutely any kind of exercise will benefit your health. If you begin walking for 30 minutes a day, even at an easy pace, you're making progress, especially if you haven't really exercised at all over the years. Walking is an excellent introduction to physical exercise and one of the best ways to keep healthy. You don't have to exercise like a professional athlete to get in shape.

Remember, start slowly. Set goals that you can achieve and get your body moving. Any kind of activity will have a positive effect. In fact, after you begin exercising routinely, you may find that you want more and more. Physical activity has a very positive effect on mental and physical health. Get going and find out for yourself.

SECTION HIGHLIGHTS
A Brief Summary of Important Points
Discussed in this Section

1. The key to losing weight and improving your diabetes involves making realistic changes to your eating and activity routine. Sensible goals—ones that are attainable—are the key to making changes that last.

2. Here's the simple breakdown of what you should do to begin losing weight.
    1. Choose a Calorie Ceiling that, when combined with exercise, will result in weight loss.
    2. Set realistic goals and make a meal plan.
    3. Stick with it.

3. Use a food diary. When you read your food diary, you have to look for patterns in order to make healthy changes. Ask yourself specific questions and come up with specific answers that identify patterns.

4. The 1-2-3 Diabetes Diet focuses on calorie counting as its method of losing weight; therefore, you'll have to set a personalized Calorie Ceiling. For a Calorie Ceiling to be effective, it needs to be lower than your current calorie intake, but high enough that you do not find yourself starving and wanting to eat everything in sight. You should always try to eat at or around your Calorie Ceiling. If you go too low, you'll end up binging. If you go over it, you'll gain weight.

5. Once you have your Calorie Ceiling set, you'll want to divide that number of calories into separate meals and snacks over the day. This is called a meal plan. Following a meal plan will guarantee that your meals contain the right nutrients, balance your blood glucose levels over time, and stay within your Calorie Ceiling. There are many ways to develop a meal plan, and you can consult with a registered dietitian to make this process easier and more personalized.

6. The easiest way to achieve a healthy diet and maintain a healthy weight begins at the grocery store and shopping the smart way. When you go to the grocery store, hit the outside aisles first. Make grocery lists before going and just purchase the items

you've put on it. Always be sure to read food labels and choose the healthiest options.

7. There are six food myths that should be busted, and here's why.

   - Eating too much fat does not make you fat, eating too many calories makes you fat.
   - Eating sugar does not give you diabetes or necessarily make your diabetes worse.
   - Fat-free foods are not guilt-free. These foods still contain calories.
   - A food that has had no sugar added may still have sugar.
   - Eating protein does not build muscle mass.
   - You do not need to eat foods in special combinations to receive a health benefit from what you've eaten.

8. For the most part, many people misunderstand carbohydrates. Dietary carbohydrate comes mostly comes in three forms: sugars, starches, and fiber. A few handy tips:

   - Choose carbohydrates that are wholesome and contain fiber.
   - Choose carbohydrates that are fresh, such as fresh fruits and vegetables.
   - Do not cover your carbohydrates in sources high in fat; this includes butter, cream, mayo and sauces.
   - Limit fried food in your diet.
   - Limit portion sizes.

9. A balanced, healthy diet revolves around eating a variety of different foods. You should never feel that certain foods are forbidden. For some of us, however, the temptation is just too great and it may prove helpful to avoid certain foods as much as possible. On the other hand, certain other foods are good for you and barely affect your Calorie Ceiling.

A Quick List

Avoid These
French fries
Fast-food sandwiches
"Americanized" Italian food
Alcoholic beverages
Ice cream and snack foods
Regular mayonnaise and
  creamy sauces

These Are Free
Water
Sugar-free and calorie-free
  drinks and snacks
Raw vegetables
Herbs and spices

---

10. Exercise is an essential part of an effective and healthy weight-loss program. A healthy amount of exercise will allow your body to burn calories faster and more efficiently. You will lose fat and build muscle. You will have more energy. Even more, you'll be able to have a higher Calorie Ceiling if you exercise. It's harder to lose weight if you're not doing anything to burn away the fat you're already carrying.

The three kinds of exercise, all of which make up an effective routine, are flexibility training, strength training, and aerobic exercise. Start slowly. Remember that doing anything to get your body moving is a step forward. Carefully check your blood glucose levels before and after (and sometimes during) exercise. Discuss your exercise plan with your health care provider.

Step Three:
Stick With It

Chapter 22

No Short Cuts! Avoiding the Temptations of Fad Diets and Magic Pills

Many of my patients often want to discuss the latest, greatest diet and see if it's right for them. Guess what. Nine times out of ten, that fad diet or magic pill isn't right for anyone. We have all seen these diets advertised, heard the testimonials, bought the diet books, and tried them ourselves. They all seem to promise the exact same things. You've heard the list a thousand times on the radio, on TV, or in magazines. Lose weight in a flash! Little to no effort required! Burn fat without exercise! Eat what you want and still lose weight! These all probably sound familiar, and you may have felt tempted in the past to see what they offer you.

Here's a news flash: they don't work—at least not over the long haul. These fad diets and magic pills offer unrealistic solutions to long-term problems. You may lose weight on some of these plans, but more often than not, you end up regaining the weight you lost in the beginning and then some. Rather than teaching a person how to eat right, fad diets and magic pills tell you to shift your behavior for a short period to lose some weight, often by excluding certain food groups.

In some cases, fad diets and magic pills can hurt you in more places than your pocketbook or wallet. They can be harmful to your health or make blood glucose control difficult. If you have diabetes, never start any diet without talking to your doctor first.

The 1-2-3 Diabetes Diet does not follow a fad. It offers a simple and healthy way to promote weight loss and good health. Like many effective and long-lasting weight-loss solutions, it also requires you to work for your rewards. Many of us cringe at the idea of working to lose weight, but it's the best way to achieve long-term health gains. Remember, anything in life that truly is important usually requires some work. And what could be more important than your health? As you learn how to follow this diet, you learn how to innately incorporate a healthy lifestyle into your daily behavior...and that's something that lasts a lifetime. To review, this is what the 1-2-3 Diabetes Diet asks of you:

- Calorie and portion control. You have to limit the food you consume. Any diet that ignores this will not work.

- Healthy food choices. Stay away from high-fat, processed, and greasy foods at home and in restaurants. Instead, choose fresh fruits and vegetables, low-fat foods, and complex carbohydrates in moderation. Once again, if the food you are about to eat looks unhealthy, fried, covered in sauces, or comes in a huge portion size, this food probably will not fit well into your healthy meal plan and should be limited.

- Exercise. Yes, your body does continually burn energy while at rest (keeping warm, breathing, etc.), but if you want to really lose weight, you need to exercise. Some people may not have truly exercised in years, so starting anything will help. Your first step should be choosing to walk more often. It's a surprisingly effective form of exercise and nearly always healthy.

Finding the Fads

Nine tips on finding out if the diet you're considering is a fad diet or a magic pill.

1. Does it promise or guarantee that you'll lose lots of weight quickly?

2. Does it tell you that you won't have to combine it with exercise?

3. Does it tell you to avoid or cut out certain food groups from your daily eating?

4. Does it offer magical results...the likes of which you'd never get from diet and exercise?

5. Do you have to buy a supplement or any other kind of special product to make weight loss happen?

6. Is there any scientific evidence supporting this weight-loss plan or does it rely on customer testimonials?

FAD DIETS

Now that you've been given a brief overview of what a fad diet is and why they should be avoided most of the time, let's look closely at two popular fads.

Low-Carbohydrate, High-Protein Diets

This type of diet has been the rage for the last few years. In this meal plan, carbohydrate intake is severely limited (cut to as close to no intake as possible) and there are no restrictions on portion size or fat intake. Commonly referred to as low-carb diets, you'll often also see them identified as high-fat diets. This is because most people on such meal plans avoid vegetables and fruit and head straight for the meat—a potent source of unhealthy fats in the American diet.

- High-fat diets can work, but only in the short term. Research has shown that some patients on high-fat, low-carb diets can lose some weight. The studies also indicate that the weight loss, like in all fad diets, is usually temporary. Part of reason seems to be that people usually lose the ability to keep up with such a diet over the long term. Ask yourself, "How long can I go without eating anything made with bread? Can I give up pizza for the rest of my life?" For many people, the novelty of the diet wears off quickly, cravings for carbohydrate take over, and the weight comes right back.

- The science behind these diets has some validity. Limiting carbohydrates, particularly refined, processed carbohydrates, is actually a good idea. Replacing these with whole-grain, complex carbohydrates and fiber instead of eliminating carbohydrate entirely from the diet is the healthiest option. I've been preaching this for a while now. Buy whole-wheat bread instead of enriched white bread and you're already making healthy progress.

- These diets partially work because of calorie restriction. Research has indicated that many people eating a high-fat diet are actually consuming fewer calories throughout the day than they did when they were eating sugary, processed foods. Eating fewer calories will certainly make you lose weight, but the health risks (particularly cardiovascular health risks, such as heart attack, clogged arteries, and the such) associated with high-fat, low-carbohydrate diets are dangerous.

- High-fat diets may be unhealthy. The jury is still out on this. In some people, the reduction in weight you get in the beginning from these diets may in fact lower your blood pressure and cholesterol. This must be balanced by the risks we already know about fat in the diet.

Slow-Carb or Glycemic Index (GI) Diets

I briefly mentioned the concept of the glycemic index in Chapter 19. The latest version of the low-carb fad is to limit foods with high glycemic indexes and eat more of those with lower glycemic indexes. When used properly and wisely, the glycemic index can be an effective meal-planning tool because it makes you think about the amount and type of carbohydrates you eat, thus helping you control your blood glucose. On the other hand, as I previously mentioned, glycemic index focuses only on the effect of a food on blood glucose levels at the expense of considering overall nutritional value. For the most part, I think you can do this on your own without relying on the glycemic index. Simply minimize the number of refined carbs you eat (junk foods, pastries, sodas) and maximize fresh, starchy carbohydrates and fiber instead of worrying about glycemic indexes. As always, watch your portion sizes.

Some Diets Do Work

There are a few healthy commercial diets available. These include point systems such as Weight Watchers and meal delivery systems such as Seattle Sutton. Both of these encourage you to use sensible calorie limits and make healthy food choices. Notice also that these products offer suggestions for adopting a healthy lifestyle that distinguish them from fad diets. They advise eating balanced meals, eating from all of the food groups, and following at least a moderate exercise routine. With this in mind, these diet plans can be very useful tools, especially if you'd like to have a guide in the process of losing weight. Personally, I think it's easier to create such a program on your own by following basic diet techniques, which will allow you to save some money.

MAGIC PILLS

The other frequent request I hear from people with diabetes is for a weight-loss pill. If you've watched TV at least once over the past few years, you've seen the ads for these. They often tell you that this magic pill will stimulate a hormone or activate some weird chemical process to encourage weight loss—with no effort on your part whatsoever. Just take the pill and it'll do all of the work for you. Guess what? If such a pill was safe, effective, and cheap, everyone would already be taking it. Magic pills make promises that cannot be kept, and even the ones that do work require watching what you eat and beginning at least a moderate exercise routine. Here is some information on the more common weight-loss pills.

1. *Appetite suppressants.* A safe, effective appetite suppressant is the Holy Grail of weight-loss medicine. Simply enough, an appetite suppressant reduces your hunger, making it easier to eat less food over the course of a day. Unfortunately, most of the currently available appetite suppressants do not meet safety requirements or work well enough. The appetite suppressants prescribed in the past were amphetamines, which stimulates the heart and blood pressure and causes a feeling of fullness. Unfortunately, these pills are unsafe and potentially addictive; many of them have been removed from the market. However, a few versions still exist. They are dangerous, and I recommend avoiding them.

    Sibutramine is a nonamphetamine medication related to some antidepressant medications that has some appetite-suppressing effects. The downside is that the weight loss associated with taking sibutramine is usually small, the pills are very expensive, it may increase heart rate and blood pressure, and the appetite effect disappears once you stop taking the medication. Still, this medication has proven effective under certain circumstances. You should consult with your doctor or health care team if you are interested in this drug.

2. *Herbal weight-loss products.* Many herbal pills claim to cause weight loss or act as appetite suppressants. Unfortunately, science rarely supports the claims of these products. If these things really worked, they would probably already be in widespread use. Drug supplements containing ephedra (also called ma huang), which has amphetamine-like qualities, were taken off the market due to health concerns in 2003. Do yourself a favor and don't get suckered into buying herbal supplements that have not been proven to work. When something that is

actually safe and effective is uncovered, medical science will be among the first to verify these claims.

3. *Fat blockers.* A drug called orlistat (brand name Xenical) blocks absorption of fat in your intestines. This is a weight-loss product that actually works. When taken with your meal, orlistat forms a chemical bond to some of the fat that you have eaten, thus keeping it from being absorbed. This means that your body metabolizes fewer calories than you have eaten (because a gram of fat contains more calories than any other nutrient), which may result in weight loss. As always, though, there are downsides. The fat that is not absorbed has to go somewhere, and major side effects of orlistat are fatty diarrhea, bloating, cramps, and gas. In addition, the drug is very expensive and not usually covered by insurance. Orlistat provides small improvements in weight loss, much of which still ultimately depends on what you are eating. Although I have seen some short-term success with orlistat, the downsides to the medication outweigh the benefits for most people.

No Short Cuts!

I hate to burst your bubble, but no short cut leads to healthy weight loss and maintenance. The best you will get from any of those advertised short cuts is short-term weight loss that leads back to weight gain. In the worst situations, misleading short cuts will cost you money, be ineffective, and possibly be dangerous to your health. It's time to realize that for weight loss to work, it will take some work. In the end, nothing is going to beat good, healthy eating habits paired with an exercise program. Properly learning how to lose weight in a healthy way—the right way—will stay with you for the rest of your life, which is a lot longer than a bottle of magic pills will last you.

Chapter 23

Hunger: Five Tips for Fighting the Red-Eyed Monster

For many people trying to lose weight, the biggest obstacle to overcome is their appetite. As we have seen, appetite is a necessary driving force we developed in nature to keep us from starving. However, when food is plentiful and cheap, as it is today, the same appetite that kept us alive in the wild can cause us to gain weight. Here are some tips to keep in mind when your appetite seems to be getting the best of you.

1. *Do not confuse hunger with other emotions.* As you studied your food diary, you probably noticed that many times you eat for reasons other than hunger. This is common. Many people eat because they're bored, depressed, or just because it's part of their routine. Learn to recognize what drives your eating and find other ways to deal with these emotions. If you feel bored, go for a walk. If you find yourself eating just because mealtime has arrived, ask yourself if you really need these calories. One good technique for fighting emotional eating is to keep the junk food out of the house. If junk food isn't available, you can't eat it when you're stressed or feeling down.

2. *Remember that hunger can be learned.* Do you ever notice how you get hungry at certain times each day? This is the body's internal clock telling you that it is time for a meal. What you will find is that it is not difficult to retrain your body. If your

body is used to a huge breakfast every morning at 8 A.M., it will expect that huge breakfast every day. As you train yourself to limit your eating throughout the day, your body will start to expect smaller meals and you will experience less hunger. In fact, less food will make you feel just as full as huge meals used to make you feel. It only takes a few days or weeks for this to work.

3. *Walk away from the table.* I don't think this is news to most people, but hunger will decrease if you wait a few minutes after you have had your meal. Evolution has trained the body to gobble down everything in sight when a meal presents itself. In survival situations, this instinct allows you to save up nutrients for later periods when food may not be plentiful. In our society, you'll always have access to food; in fact, we have access to an excess of food. Eat a reasonably sized meal, limit second helpings, and move away from the food. For the most part, within a few minutes you will feel full and satisfied after a light meal and be able to avoid overeating.

4. *Fight hunger urges with low-calorie, filling snacks.* Some of these are discussed in Chapter 20. When hunger strikes, try to eat a small piece of fruit and a glass of water. A small, healthy snack can usually stave off most hunger attacks. Also, many people can confuse the sensations of thirst with hunger. So if you're feeling really sluggish and hungry, try drinking some water first.

5. *Be prepared for nights and the TV.* Many people have the greatest problems controlling their eating habits in the evening or night. This is when most of us are at home, and food is part of the relaxation process. In addition, many of us feel we deserve a reward for a hard day of work, especially when relaxing in front of the TV. Unfortunately, these rewarding snack times are often filled with fatty, processed foods and empty calories. This is our national bad habit. How can we break this bad habit? By being prepared. You shouldn't be surprised when the late-night munchies hit, especially if it happens every night. Be ready for it. Get the junk food out of the house. Come up with healthy snack options, such as fruit, raw vegetables, or healthy snack crackers that you can prepare ahead of time so they're ready when you want them. Better yet, find something else to do to keep your mind off food and avoid unnecessary snacking. Take a walk, read to your kids, or call a friend. Don't give in; you'll feel better for it in the long run.

Chapter 24
Social Pressure

We should address something that not many people want to bring up when it comes to weight loss, especially for people with diabetes. As our society becomes more overweight and less healthy in general, those who are trying to lose weight often find themselves surrounded by people who are not very healthy themselves. Overeating and unhealthy lifestyles often run in the family and not just with one individual in that family. This can lead to some ugly situations that you may have already experienced. I'm referring to the social pressures and unintentional sabotage that can come from well-meaning friends and loved ones when you begin to lead your new health-focused lifestyle.

Let's put this into more practical terms. When people begin dieting and exercising, they will often have jokes directed at them or loving concern. If you go to a restaurant and order a salad with dressing on the side instead of your normal hamburger, you may get a few snide remarks from friends and family. If you're sitting down to eat dinner at home and don't get your normal second serving, your family may ask what's wrong and try to force you to eat more. After all, a second serving is what you've always had—maybe there's something wrong with you.

Thinking about your health and taking action may also draw some grumbles from those close to you who don't feel they need to change. If you start to park farther away from the store so you can get some walking in, others in the car may complain. If exercise starts to get in the way of old routines, such as sitting in front of the TV all night, people may try to talk you into staying in and avoiding exercise. If your Sunday football game snacks suddenly become healthy treats rather than the old fat-laden goodies they used to be, people may resent that.

Why do people act like this? There are many reasons. Some people feel embarrassed when someone around them starts trying to lose weight because it makes them feel like they should lose weight as well. If you start to lose weight and a close friend or family member becomes self-conscious about his or her own weight, that person may try to convince you to stop changing your lifestyle. After all, this is easier than having to change theirs. Some research has even shown that parents of overweight children do not encourage weight loss in their children because it would mean that they'd have to lose weight as well.

These are sad facts, but often they can be true. This tendency from the people we love and trust most makes a difficult task even harder. You're going to be working hard enough to control your own urges and desires, but with some people, you will also have to contend with them urging you to go back to your old ways. You will absolutely have to resist this. After all, this isn't just about looking better—your health is at stake.

Here are some tips for countering social pressure.

- *Tell them why you're doing this.* Make sure that these people understand why you are making changes to your lifestyle. Tell them about your diabetes and the risks that come with it. Your health and future livelihood are at stake here. Ensuring a long life will require sacrifices and changes now. Honesty, as they say, is the best policy, and coming up straight with your friends and loved ones about diabetes and weight loss will often get the best response. The people who are truly important to your life should realize that pressuring you to jeopardize your health isn't very kind.

- *Inform them that these changes are permanent and they'll need to get used to them.* Sometimes people may just need to see that you are serious about your new lifestyle changes and that's all they need to stop pressuring you. Make it clear that joking and nagging are unappreciated and counterproductive. In fact, these activities will change nothing about your new lifestyle, so it's better for everyone to just accept it and move on.

- *Quietly continue with your plan and ignore the comments.* This tactic works for some people, but not for many. It may seem like the simple solution to social pressure, but in reality, when our closest friends and family confront us mercilessly about lifestyle changes, we tend to listen. After all, these people are closest to us—we trust and value their thoughts and opinions.

It is better to talk with your loved ones about your decision to change your lifestyle. They may become supportive and helpful in your new plan, and some of them may even join you.

- *Tell them that by cheating your diet and exercise plan, you're only cheating yourself, not your doctor.* This is an excuse I often hear: "Come on, just eat the burger and fries, your doctor won't know." No, your doctor won't know, but your body will. Your doctor isn't going to gain weight and develop diabetes complications if you continue to eat poorly, but you might. Make sure that the people pressuring you to cheat know this as well.

- *Think of yourself as a healthy example.* Often times, the people who rib you the most are the ones who could most benefit from a healthy lifestyle as well. If this is someone in your family, think of your change for the better as you leading by example. Perhaps this will inspire someone close to you to start paying better attention to their own health. If so, now you have a partner in this challenge and that always makes any task easier.

- *Join a support group.* If the social pressure becomes overwhelming and none of the approaches described here seem to work, think about joining a support group. They provide peer support in many ways, and joining such a group and describing your problems may help. Some of the members may provide some helpful advice, and you will likely see that you're not alone in your troubles and worries. In addition to this topic, support groups can help you deal with your diabetes in so many other ways. If you are familiar and comfortable with the Internet, you can search for online message boards for people with diabetes. The American Diabetes Association has a pretty nice one available at *www.diabetes.org.*

- *Consult with your doctor or health care team.* As always, your doctor and health care team should be around to provide helpful support when it is necessary. Though you may not feel that the topic of social pressure falls under their area of knowledge, you should bring it up with them if it is a serious issue that concerns you. Social pressure such as this can affect your blood glucose levels (be it through eating habits or just anxiety), and you should feel comfortable enough with your health care providers to mention it.

- *Remember that you are the first priority right now.* This may seem selfish, especially if other people (such as your family or close friends) rely on you, but you need to take care of yourself. If you're not around because you don't take care of your diabetes, who will take care of the people who need you? Taking care of yourself should be your first priority when it comes to losing weight, exercising, and monitoring your diabetes.

Chapter 25
Healthy Hints: Surviving Restaurant Menus

You've put together a meal plan, started exercising, and watched what you buy at the grocery store. By now, you should have a pretty good idea of what your blood glucose goals are, and you've found a way to lose weight. That's a lot to take on, but now you're going to have to face the toughest challenge in a weight-loss plan—eating at restaurants. This is no easy task. American restaurants provide gigantic portions and often-unhealthy food.

Still, eating a healthy meal at a restaurant isn't impossible, and it can be done at most places, including some fast-food restaurants, chain restaurants, and your favorite local places. What you may not like, however, is the fact that eating a healthy meal at these restaurants will require you to give up some of your favorite dishes in exchange for healthier ones. In addition, going out to eat will require planning, which doesn't make going to a restaurant the quick and easy pleasure it once was.

HOW TO HANDLE RESTAURANTS

Do you remember when you evaluated your eating habits? You probably noticed you were eating out a lot. This is common. Americans eat out at restaurants more now than they ever have. In order to combat the effects eating out has on our overall health, we need to know how eating at restaurants affects us personally. Here is a list of questions you should ask yourself when considering the role restaurants have in your life.

- *How often do I eat out?*

   The more often you eat meals at restaurants (or take-out, fast food, whatever), the less control you have over what you're eating. It's easy to avoid thinking about the calories and fat grams in the food you eat at restaurants because it normally requires some effort to find that information. Most of us often tell ourselves not to worry about the details, order what we want, and enjoy the food.

   So, when you think about your habits with eating out, consider how often you eat meals away from home. Think about how many meals that adds up to over the course of a week or month. Compare weekday patterns with those on weekends.

- *Normally, which meals do I eat away from home?*

   Much like the question above, understanding how often you eat out can show you where to improve your diet with healthier options. Look for trends. Do you just eat lunch at restaurants? Do you eat all of your meals out? Knowing these things about yourself is important.

- *Why do I eat at restaurants?*

   For so long, eating out at restaurants has been seen as a special event, something we do to celebrate. You go out to eat to when someone gets a promotion or has a birthday or anniversary—just about any special event. This trend still stands, but with our busy lifestyles, eating out has become a habit. It's easier to let someone else cook for you, and it takes less time. Think about why you eat out. Is it because it is quick and convenient? Do you hate the idea of cooking or even entering your kitchen? Are restaurants where you always go for social gatherings? Do restaurants provide better food than you think you can cook at home? Restaurants can continue to be an important part of your new healthy lifestyle, but you'll need to make plans when eating out and remove some of your reliance on them as your only source of meals.

- *At what kinds of restaurants do I eat?*

   Restaurants come in all shapes and sizes. Some offer all-you-can-eat buffets, some are counter-service, fast-food types, and others are extensive chains that offer the same menu in every location. Restaurants can be diners, local favorites, or expensive and fancy establishments. There is no end to where you can order food, and that's a wonderful thing about life. However, the choices you make in where you eat can affect your weight and your diabetes. By knowing where you like to eat, you can make changes to your meal plan to fit in foods at those places. You'll also know where your extra calories are coming from.

- *What kinds of foods do I eat at restaurants? How big are the portion sizes I tend to order?*
  High-fat foods and gigantic portions are the killers you'll find in any restaurant, whether it's a really long sub sandwich or a loaded platter of ribs, fries, and some vegetables. Most of the time, you're usually eating enough food for two or even three people.

Answering these questions is the first step toward healthier restaurant eating. Much like with your food diary, you're looking for patterns that you can change for the better. If you have a habit of getting the biggest burger at a fast-food restaurant every day for lunch, that's something you'll want to tackle with your meal plan. If you find that you eat out most of the time because you don't have enough food at home, think about what you can do to motivate yourself out to the grocery store and into your own kitchen. Our restaurant habit can be easily addressed; it's just that making these changes will take some investigation, some work, and some dedication.

STRATEGIES FOR SUCCESS

Eating out can be filled with challenges and pitfalls. Often, a meal at a fast-food restaurant will provide enough fat and calories to feed one person for an entire day. The meal you get from a family chain restaurant is often enough to feed a small family.

You may think the odds are stacked against you, but they're not. Here are several tips on how to plan your restaurant attack and get out without taking in too many calories. Keep in mind that when you begin your meal plan and exercise program, it may be in your best interest to really cut down on restaurants or avoid them altogether, simply to remove the temptation to overeat.

Order Up!

If you eat out often, find ways to follow your meal plan as much as possible. Pick a restaurant with a variety of choices. This will increase your chances of finding the foods you want. Remember that when you eat out, you should order only what you need and want. Know how to make changes in your meal plan in case the restaurant doesn't have just what you want.

Some restaurants will better meet your personal needs if you phone ahead or do some planning online. Many large restaurants have websites that post their menu. Some of the restaurant chains also provide the nutritional information of many of their dishes.

If you enjoy the healthy choices on a restaurant's menu, you should let the management know. If you want more low-calorie, low-cholesterol choices, say so. Restaurants, just like any other business, offer what their customers want, and they only know what you want if you tell them.

Ordering Tips

- If you don't know what's in a dish or don't know the serving size, ask your server.
- Try to eat the same portion size as you would at home. If the serving size is larger, share some with your dining partner or take the extra portion home.
- Eat slowly.
- Ask for fish or meat broiled and with no extra butter.
- Order your baked potato plain and top it with a teaspoon of margarine (or a healthy butter substitute) or low-calorie sour cream and/or vegetables from the salad bar.
- Ask for sauces, gravy, and salad dressings on the side. Try dipping your fork in the salad dressing and then spear a piece of lettuce. Another option is to add a teaspoon of dressing at a time to your salad. You'll use less this way.
- Order foods that are not breaded or fried because these cooking methods add calories. If your food comes breaded, peel off the outer coating.
- Read the menu creatively. Order a fruit cup for an appetizer or the breakfast melon for dessert. Instead of a dinner meal, combine a salad with a low-fat appetizer.
- Ask for healthier substitutions. Instead of French fries, request a double order of a vegetable. If you can't get a substitute, just ask that the high-fat food be left off your order.
- Ask for low-calorie items, such as salad dressings, even if they're not on the menu. Vinegar and a dash of oil or a squeeze of lemon are better choices than high-fat dressings, such as ranch and bleu cheese.
- Limit your alcoholic drinks; they add calories but no nutrition to your meal.

Timing Your Meals

If you take diabetes pills or insulin shots, think about when you'll eat as well as what you'll eat. You can avoid diabetes problems by planning.

- If you're eating out with others, ask them to eat at your usual time so that it doesn't require that you change the timing of your medications.

- Plan your meals so that you won't be kept waiting for a table when you need to be eating.

- Make reservations and be on time. Avoid the times when the restaurant is busiest so that you won't have to wait.

- Ask whether personalized dishes will take extra time to prepare.

- If your lunch or dinner is going to be later than usual, eat your after-meal snack before dinner to hold you over.

Conquering Fast Food

Just because you have diabetes doesn't mean that you can never eat fast food ever again. But you need to know exactly what you are ordering and plan ahead. Keep the ground rules of good nutrition in mind. Eat a variety of foods in moderate amounts, limit the amount of fat you eat, and watch the amount of salt in food. Follow the guidelines you've worked out with your doctor or registered dietitian.

What you order is the key to healthy fast-food meals. It's easy to eat an entire day's worth of fat, salt, and calories in just one meal. On the other hand, you can also make wise choices and eat a relatively healthy meal. Here some tips to help you keep fast food within your Calorie Ceiling.

- Know that an average fast-food meal can run as high as 1,000 calories or more and raise your blood glucose above your target range.

- Know the nutritional value of the foods you order. Although there are some good choices, most fast-food items are high in fat and calories. Researching the restaurant's menu beforehand can be helpful in planning what you are going to order.

- If you're having fast food for one meal, let your other meals that day contain healthier foods, such as fruits and vegetables.

- Think about how your food will be cooked. Chicken and fish can be good choices, but not if they are breaded and deep fried.

Approaching the Menu

There are healthy foods in restaurants. Sometimes, though, it may feel like they're hidden. Here are some suggestions on how to read menus and make sure the food you are ordering is the healthiest option.

- Look for keywords on the menu, such as *jumbo, giant, deluxe, super size, family style, heaping,* and *generous.* Large portions mean more calories. They also mean more fat, cholesterol, and salt. Order a regular or junior-sized meal instead.

- Choose grilled or broiled sandwiches with lean meats, such as lean roast beef, turkey or chicken breast, or lean ham. Order items plain, without toppings, rich sauces, or mayonnaise. Add flavor with mustard, lettuce, tomato, and onion.

- Skip croissants or biscuits; they are surprisingly high in calories and fat. Eat your sandwiches on a bun, bread, or English muffin and save yourself some calories and fat.

- Stay away from double, triple, and mega-burgers or hot dogs with cheese, chili, or sauces. Cheese carries an extra 100 calories per ounce, as well as added fat and sodium. Extra burger patties can carry even more calories, fat, and sodium than extra cheese.

- Be careful of the salad bar. Just about everyone agrees that the salad bar is a healthy choice, as long as you are wise about what you put on your salad. The same goes for salads that you order off of menus; some of them can have more calories and fat than a sandwich. A salad with a large hunk of fried chicken and handful of cheese sitting on top is not healthy just because it's a salad. The lettuce does not cancel out the calorie-rich dressing. Check the nutritional information, if available. Be careful of high-fat toppers like creamy dressings, croutons (yep, croutons), cheese, and bacon bits. You should also limit salad bar items that come with a lot of mayonnaise, including potato salad, macaroni salad, chicken salad, and tuna salad. To keep the taste, fill your salad with healthy vegetables, such as carrots, peppers, onion, celery, broccoli, cauliflower, spinach, and tomatoes.

- Order bean burritos, soft tacos, fajitas, and other non-fried items when eating Mexican meals. Whenever possible, choose chicken over beef and cut down on refried beans. Better yet, ask your server if you can have beans that aren't refried. Pile on extra lettuce, tomatoes, and salsa, but go easy on the cheese, sour cream, and guacamole. Be careful to watch out for deep-fried taco salad shells. A taco salad can have more than 1,000 calories!

- Believe it or not, pizza can be a good fast food choice. Go for thin crust with vegetable toppings. Limit yourself to one or two slices. Meat and extra cheese add calories, fat, and sodium, so you should be careful what you have on it.

- End your meal with a small cone of fat-free frozen yogurt (but remember that just because it is fat-free doesn't mean it's calorie-free). Better still, have a piece of fresh fruit. Ices, sorbets, and sherbets have less fat and fewer calories than ice cream, but are full of sugar. They can send your blood glucose too high if you don't work the extra carbohydrate into your meal plan.

- Be aware of deceptive "healthy" foods. Fat-free muffins for breakfast may seem healthier than that fast-food sandwich, but they still have their downside. Fat-free muffins can have plenty of sugar. Skinless fried chicken can have almost as much fat as the regular kind. Chinese food may seem like a healthy choice, but many dishes are deep fried or high in fat and sodium, especially in the sauces. Do your research and be aware of what you eat.

Chapter 26
Assessing Your Progress

So you've followed the steps in this book. You've examined your eating habits, made changes, and come up with a meal plan that works for you. Now it's time to look at your progress. After all, how else can you identify and understand your strengths and weaknesses if you don't keep track of where you've been and where you're going? Knowing which areas need improvement helps you adjust your meal plan and lifestyle over time, ensuring even more progress. Start your assessment by evaluating yourself on the following points.

1. *Blood glucose control.* The most important factor in the treatment of diabetes is proper blood glucose control. You should already be checking your blood glucose levels several times a day. Your doctor or health care team should also be conducting A1C checks at least once or twice a year. If your numbers are not meeting your target numbers, you should probably make some adjustments to your plan. Maybe you need to make more changes to your meal plan, or you need new medication. Generally, healthy eating, exercise, and weight loss should result in lower blood glucose levels, so if you're not seeing any improvement over time, you should meet with your doctor, health care team, or a dietitian to discuss possible solutions.

Keep This in Mind

Though a self-assessment should involve examining changes in your blood glucose levels over the period between self-assessments, you definitely need to check your blood glucose frequently and regularly, as advised by your health care provider. Avoiding your blood glucose levels for whatever reason is a surefire way to negatively affect your diabetes. Checking your blood glucose is the first and most important step in taking care of your diabetes.

2. *Weight.* As we discussed early on in Chapter 2, an important tool is your personal scale. You should try to check your weight at least two or three times a week, if not more often. A large part of the 1-2-3 Diabetes Diet is dedicated to weight control and weight loss precisely because it is such a struggle for most people, especially those with type 2 diabetes. No one ever said weight loss was going to be easy to master, but as we have seen, the worst thing you can do is ignore your waistline. If your weight is not under control, you and your health care team need to continue to address this issue.

3. *Overall health.* In many ways, your overall fitness represents your overall health. How do you feel overall? As your health improves and your blood glucose and weight get under control, you should feel better. This feeling will normally carry through to other parts of your life: you'll feel better emotionally, you'll have more energy, and you'll want to do more things. Do you have more energy? Can you get around easier? Is physical activity less tiring than it used to be? Are you happy with how you look and feel? As your overall health improves, you should be able to say yes to all of these questions. If not, definitely bring this up with your health care team and see what else they can suggest. A major goal of health care, after all, is getting you to feel better.

Q&A

How often should I do a self-assessment?

That's a good question. When you first begin the 1-2-3 Diabetes Diet, aim for a self-assessment twice a week, more often if you feel you need it. Keep in mind that you're not going to see dramatic results right away. In fact, from day to day, change should be moderate and small. After all, you're shooting for a weight loss of one to two pounds a week. However, over the span of a few weeks, you should begin to notice a greater change. Remember that the healthy way to lose weight is to lose it gradually while getting more fit. As you build muscle, which weighs more than fat, it will look like your weight loss is slowing down but you'll notice a difference in your body shape.

As time passes, you probably won't need to self-evaluate as frequently, probably just a few times a month. You will become more accustomed to knowing whether you are making progress or not. In the beginning, use the self-assessment to encourage yourself and to make sure that you set off on the right track. Self-assessment will allow you to catch any straying from the start.

WHAT IF THINGS AREN'T GOING WELL?

What do you do if your self-assessment shows a lack of progress or even movement in the wrong direction? First, make sure your expectations of the self-assessment are not too high. If you find that you've lost two pounds, but you thought you worked hard enough to lose five pounds, then the hard truth is that you now know how much effort it will take to lose just two pounds a week. And remember that losing two pounds in a week is great! Over a year that's 104 pounds. Set reasonable and realistic goals for yourself and do the best you can. Your self-assessments can be reassuring and encouraging, but they may not always tell you exactly what you want to hear.

However, there are the situations where things clearly aren't going as well. What if after the first self-assessment, you find that you've gained weight or your blood glucose levels have steadily gotten higher? What do you do in these situations? Once again, good health doesn't have any easy answers, but I'll describe a few places where you can start.

1. *Talk to your health providers.* Your doctor and health care team should be available to help you when you need it. Consult with them about the results of your lifestyle changes and see what they say. Remember that when it comes to your health, you are the customer in a health care setting, and you should expect to see a reasonable response to your requests for help. If you feel you are not getting good answers about your health from your providers, it is time to find some new ones.

2. *Every day is a new start.* Just because your first shot at getting healthy hasn't gone as planned doesn't mean that you will never succeed. In fact, it often takes people several serious attempts at lifestyle change before it sticks. Every morning that you wake up is a new chance to eat right, exercise, and get healthy. Keep the positive attitude and positive things will happen.

3. *Seek support from other people with diabetes.* Many communities have diabetes support groups. Joining these groups is an excellent way to learn more and meet others struggling with the same issues. It is helpful to see others facing the same problems you face, and you can gain valuable advice and support from people who have dealt with the same issues you are currently having. The more people who take part in your goal of getting healthy, the more likely that you will succeed. After all, it's one thing to let yourself down, but it's so much

harder when you let down a group of people rooting for your success.

4. *Do some research.* I mentioned earlier that this should not be the only diabetes book you own. Not by a long shot. There is simply too much to know, and the more you know about health, the easier it is to get healthy. There are a variety of good books about diabetes and weight loss available. Read them. You can also use the Internet to find resources, but be careful; not everything you read on the Internet is true. Make sure the information is coming from credible sources and that claims are backed by science. Just because someone says something on a message board doesn't mean it's a good idea.

5. *Don't give up.* Nothing is more important than your health. Whatever you do, keep trying. You may feel that this is a battle between you, your body, and diabetes. More often than not, adopting a healthy lifestyle is a battle of willpower and dedication. Keep a positive attitude! You can do it!

Chapter 27

Five Ways to Boost Your Metabolism (and Four of Them Don't Involve Exercise)

If you burn more calories than you take in, you lose weight. You've heard this again and again, and just about any reliable weight-loss plan will say the exact same thing. Up to this point, we have concentrated on ways to control calorie intake. The other important part to losing weight, however, is burning more calories. The more calories you burn, the more calories you can eat without gaining weight. Exercise is the quickest and easiest way to do this. However, there are other ways to boost your metabolism and burn more calories. Here are five ways to boost metabolism, and four of them don't require exercise.

1. *Exercise.* The benefits of exercise are well known. Not only does exercise burn calories and boost your metabolism, exercise offers other health benefits. Aside from weight loss, exercise lessens insulin resistance, making your diabetes medications work better and your blood glucose levels easier to control. Blood pressure, cholesterol levels, and cardiovascular function can also improve with regular exercise.

2. *Move.* Okay, technically we are still talking about exercise, but let's not call it that. Studies have shown that small changes in your lifestyle can have a big impact. If I can't talk you into 20 minutes on the treadmill, can I at least get you to turn off the

TV and move around a bit? Walk up a few flights of stairs instead of the elevator. Take an evening walk. Park farther away in the parking lot and burn a few calories. The more you move the better, and anything is better than nothing.

3. *Do not starve yourself.* Fasting and starvation can actually work against weight loss. When your calorie intake gets too low, your body enters starvation mode and attempts to conserve the body stores. The body does this by slowing your metabolism. As a result, weight loss slows to almost nothing. Thus, starvation dieting is very often unsuccessful. It's also dangerous. When the body runs out of fuel from the food you eat, it begins to burn fat and then moves on to your muscle. If you start losing muscle mass due to starvation, organ damage may result. Avoid this starvation mode and eat at your Calorie Ceiling, not drastically below it.

4. *Eat throughout the day.* This sounds weird, doesn't it? For most of this book I've been telling you to eat less. I still am. You should always stay underneath your Calorie Ceiling. However, if you spread those calories out throughout the day instead of bunching them into two or three meals, you can actually boost your metabolism. It sounds backward, but eating more often is actually the easiest way to eat less. Doing this helps you avoid between-meal hunger (which can lead to overeating) and provides a steady source of fuel that keeps your metabolism up and provides you with more energy. Try it; instead of breaking your Calorie Ceiling down into three meals, break it down into four or five. You won't be getting as much at one meal, but it can be comforting to know that your next meal is only a couple of hours away.

5. *Use temperature to your advantage.* One of the major ways the body burns calories is by maintaining your body's internal temperature, a critical function for staying alive. More calories are burned when you are exposed to warm or cool conditions. One way to take advantage of this is to subject yourself to mild temperature extremes. Keep your surroundings a little cooler in the winter and a little warmer in the summer and you will burn a few extra calories with no work whatsoever.

Chapter 28

Other Meal-Planning Options: Carb Counting, Fat Grams, and Exchange Lists

I've based the 1-2-3 Diabetes Diet on counting calories and exercise. Both will help you lose weight, which will automatically help your diabetes. But if you want to get your glucose levels under better control, you'll need to do more, especially if you are using insulin. To better manage your blood glucose levels and offset the development of complications, you should try counting carbohydrates. Counting fat grams and using exchange lists can also help you lose weight and maintain good diabetes care. I'll describe each one briefly in this chapter, but if you intend to pursue any of these options further, you can find some handy guides published by the American Diabetes Association, including the *Complete Guide to Carb Counting, 2nd edition,* and the *Exchange List for Meal Planning,* co-published with the American Dietetic Association.

COUNTING CARBOHYDRATE

We have already seen that eating carbohydrate has the biggest effect on your blood glucose levels. We also know that carbohydrate is one of the essential forms of energy we receive from the foods we eat. Therefore, carbohydrate counting is a popular and successful method of managing diet and controlling diabetes. Generally, your best bet in starting a carbohydrate-counting program will require seeing a registered dietitian beforehand.

To use carbohydrate counting, you must know the total carbohydrate amount you're allowed to eat for the day. This is sort of like a Carbohydrate Ceiling. A registered dietitian can help you find this number and work with you in creating a meal plan based on how much you normally eat, as well as your physical activity, medications, and lifestyle. When you begin this kind of meal plan, you will need to become familiar with the carbohydrate content in foods. Because we find carbohydrate in many foods, such as grains, vegetables, fruits, milk, and table sugar, it is important to learn as much as possible about the foods you eat.

Carbohydrate counting can provide some advantages over other meal-planning approaches. Some people feel that focusing on only one nutrient make this system easier. With the focus on carbohydrate, food and insulin can be matched more precisely. Matching food and insulin increases flexibility in meal and snack times. This can be particularly helpful when your appetite varies or your schedule changes. Also, insulin can be matched to carbohydrate eaten at specific times during the day, which is especially helpful for people with type 1 diabetes.

On the other hand, carbohydrate counting does come with one disadvantage. If you spend all of your time focusing on carbohydrate content alone, you can lose track of the other nutrients you're eating. Many foods contain no carbs at all, but are loaded with fat and calories. For example, if you just count the carbohydrate in a steak (almost none) but don't think about the other nutrients, you may end up with a lot more fat and calories in your diet than you planned. Ignoring important issues like this may make your meal plan counterproductive (you gain weight) and unhealthy (the increased disease risk of a high-fat diet).

What Am I Counting?

Sometimes, the task of counting carbohydrates is made easier by having people count carbohydrate choices. This term describes a single, 15-gram serving of carbohydrate. Using this standard measure makes carbohydrate counting easy because you won't have to use a calculator or keep detailed logs of the carbohydrate content of the foods you've eaten. You'll also become more familiar with what a 15-gram serving of carbohydrate looks like, making this meal plan even easier to follow.

I strongly recommend meeting with a registered dietitian (see Chapter 29) before beginning a carbohydrate-counting plan, but here's a short list of what some carbohydrate allotments are for certain diet plans.

1,500-calorie meal plan	12 Carbohydrate choices
1,800-calorie meal plan	14 Carbohydrate choices
2,000-calorie meal plan	16 Carbohydrate choices

COUNTING FAT GRAMS

This method of dieting is probably familiar to you. After all, counting fat has been preached by health professionals for some time now. Unfortunately, it doesn't seem to have a very good track record. Many people have had bad luck with simply counting fat, probably because they don't also count calories. There are many high-calorie, fat-free foods available that can lead to weight gain, such as soda, candy, fat-free chips, fat-free ice-cream, and more. Even worse, there was a common myth for a long time that if something didn't have fat, you could eat as much as you want, which is simply not true.

This isn't to say that counting fat grams is all bad. There are some benefits to fat-counting diets. Because fat contains so many more calories than any other nutrient, lowering the amount you eat can automatically lower your calorie intake, so long as those calories aren't replaced by other, unhealthy foods. It is also simple and provides quite a bit of flexibility and control over your food choices. With fat-gram counting, you will usually improve the overall quality of your food choices because you will tend to select lower-fat foods, such as fruits, vegetables, grains, and low-fat dairy products. Like carbohydrate counting, you are focusing on only one nutrient. This can be appealing when weight loss is the primary goal and other approaches have not worked.

Still, simply counting fat grams may not be the best choice for people with diabetes. For sure, you will want to limit the amount of fat you eat, especially saturated fats and *trans*-fats. But without considering calories and also making healthy choices, fat-gram counting is not a sure-fire weight loss option. Plus, it does not take into consideration the foods that may affect your blood glucose. Therefore, your blood glucose values may be inconsistent.

USING EXCHANGE LISTS

Many health professionals and people with diabetes swear by exchange lists, a versatile and healthy meal-planning tool. It can take some time to become familiar with using exchanges in your daily meals, but after awhile, it becomes easier and easier.

Here's how exchange lists work. The system groups foods with similar nutritional values into lists. Each serving of food in that list has about the same number of calories, carbohydrate, protein, and fat as a serving of the other foods in the same list. Therefore, an exchange describes not only what kind of food you can eat, but also the serving size. You can exchange any food on a list for another food in that same list. Therefore, by using exchanges, people with diabetes can almost guarantee that their meals will be nutritious and balanced.

There are several different exchange lists, but they are broken down into three very large groups: carbohydrate, meat and meat substitutes, and fat. These three groups are broken down further into lists that are more specific. For example, the carbohydrate list includes starch exchanges, fruit exchanges, milk exchanges, other carbohydrate exchanges, and nonstarchy vegetable exchanges. Three other lists group foods that don't fall into those above: free foods, combination foods, and fast foods. One thing to note is that a single exchange of a food doesn't necessarily represent a single serving. The typical serving size of a particular food may add up to as many as five exchanges.

To follow an exchange-list meal plan, you'll definitely need to meet with a registered dietitian. He or she will work with you to set up a meal plan that breaks down your daily eating into a group of exchanges. For example, you may be told that your daily meal plan will consist of the following exchanges: 7 starch, 4 fruit, 3 milk, 4 nonstarchy vegetables, 6 lean meats, and 7 fats. You can select any foods you want from the exchanges provided, but cannot exceed the number given to you and should avoid using fewer exchanges than those allotted. You will also need to buy a guide to exchange lists.

The advantage to using exchange lists is that it focuses on overall nutrition. Because you get to eat many different foods and exchanges cover almost all of them, your meal plan emphasizes many different nutrients. This system also encourages consistency in the timing and amount of your meals and snacks. Exchange lists also help teach you how to calculate the nutritional content of the foods you eat, which might benefit those using carbohydrate counting. A carbohydrate exchange contains about 15 grams of carbohydrate, which is the same as the carbohydrate choice described above.

On the other hand, learning how to use exchange lists can be time consuming, difficult, and frustrating. A registered dietitian is a perfect guide to learning about exchange lists. You'll also have to learn how to calculate the exchange value for a food not described in the exchange lists. Still, some food companies have started including the exchange value for the food on its food label, which is very handy for beginners and people on the move.

Chapter 29
Do I Need a
Registered Dietitian?

You've gotten this far with the 1-2-3 Diabetes Diet, but what if things aren't quite working as you like or if you need more help putting together meal plans? Perhaps you're losing weight, but your blood glucose levels aren't predictable. If problems start to arise, you may find it very helpful to see a registered dietitian (RD).

An RD is trained in nutrition and has passed a national exam. An RD may also have a master's degree and may be a Certified Diabetes Educator (CDE). You want to be sure to work with an RD who has training and experience with diabetes.

A dietitian can help you figure out your food needs based on your desired weight, lifestyle, medication, and other health goals (such as lowering blood fat levels or blood pressure). Even if you've had diabetes for many years, a visit to the dietitian can help. For one thing, our food needs change as we get older. Nutrition guidelines for people with diabetes also change from time to time, and an RD can keep your diet up to date with the latest research.

Dietitians can also help you learn how

- the foods you eat affect your blood sugar and blood fat levels
- to balance food with medications and activity
- to read food labels
- to make a sick-day meal plan
- to plan meals
- to plan for eating out and special events

- to include ethnic or foreign foods into your meals

- to find good cookbooks

- to make food substitutions

Most of the time, your doctor will be able to recommend an RD if he or she does not have one on staff. If you'd like to find one on your own, you can search for one in your area by visiting the American Dietetic Association's website (*http://www.eatright.org*).

SECTION HIGHLIGHTS
A Brief Summary of Important Points
Discussed in this Section

1. There are no true short cuts to losing weight, no matter what you see or hear in advertisements. Some of the short cuts these magic pills and fad diets propose can be dangerous to people with diabetes. Keep an eye out for these overrated products and plans, so you don't fall victim to their false promises. On the other hand, you can avoid them altogether and lose weight the healthy way—by following the 1-2-3 Diabetes Diet.

2. Fighting your appetite or hunger will be a key factor in losing weight effectively. When you begin your meal plan and follow your Calorie Ceiling, you will no doubt feel hungry at first. Fighting the urge to eat until you feel stuffed will be difficult, but it's not an impossible task. Here are some tips in overcoming your hunger.

   - Do not confuse hunger with other emotions.
   - Remember that hunger can be learned.
   - Walk away from the table when you're finished eating.
   - Fight hunger urges with low-calorie, filling snacks.
   - Be prepared for nights and the TV.

3. It's an unfortunate fact, but sometimes a person's closest loved ones are the most critical when he or she decides to make significant lifestyle changes. Here are some tips for defusing peer pressure and seeking help.

   - Tell them why you're doing this.
   - Inform them that these changes are permanent and to get used to them.
   - Quietly continue with your plan and ignore the comments.
   - Tell them that by cheating your diet and exercise plan, you're only cheating yourself, not your doctor.
   - Think of yourself as a healthy example.
   - Join a support group.
   - Consult with your doctor or health care team.
   - Remember that you are the first priority right now.

4. One of the most challenging tasks of getting on a meal plan and losing weight is facing the ordeals of eating out. Generally, it's better to avoid eating out as much as possible when beginning a new meal plan, simply to remove temptation. However, it is quite possible to have healthy meals when eating out, wherever you decide to eat.

In many ways, the most successful strategies for approaching eating in restaurants are those that also apply to selecting which foods you'll eat at home—planning, research, and self-control. If you can make wise choices, you'll enjoy eating out as much as you did before you began watching what you eat.

5. The only way you'll really know whether the 1-2-3 Diabetes Diet is working for you is by assessing your progress. When conducting a self-assessment, you need to consider your blood glucose levels, weight, and overall health. Look for changes over time and see if you are making progress.

   If your self-assessments are showing little to no progress, it may help to follow these tips:

   • Talk to your health providers.
   • Remember that every day is a new start.
   • Seek support from other people with diabetes.
   • Do some research.
   • Don't give up.

6. Exercise isn't the only way to give your metabolism a little boost and burn away some extra calories. Here are some other ways.

   • Get moving (technically exercise, but any amount of movement helps).
   • Do not starve yourself.
   • Eat less food more often throughout the day.
   • Use temperature to your advantage.

7. As you begin to hit your weight-loss goals and become familiar with the concepts of diet and exercise, it may be time to take on more advanced techniques that will further improve your blood glucose levels. These new techniques include counting carbohydrates, counting fat grams, and using exchange lists. Of these, the first and last are probably the most helpful, and they'll be easier to master after you've become capable at counting calories.

8. If you feel lost or like you could use some help in losing weight, always consider consulting with a registered dietitian (RD). RDs are educated in nutrition and many specialize in treating people with diabetes. They can help you put together strong meal plans and help you troubleshoot your diet plan if it is not working as well as you'd expected. Ask your doctor for a referral or contact the American Dietetic Association.

Appendix
Helpful Resources

This is a long road you've undertaken, but it will have very positive effects on your health and general well-being. In the long term, you may find that you need some extra information or help, so here are some helpful diabetes resources. This list comes far short of being comprehensive, but it should provide a good starting point.

WEBSITES

When it comes to putting quick and easy information at your fingertips, nothing works better than the Internet. But remember to be selective about the information you find here. Not everything is trustworthy. Websites run by long-standing, national organizations are usually your best bet. Websites trying to sell you something are generally not to be trusted.

Many people feel intimidated by the Internet, and if you're one of those people, you should at least try to visit these websites and see what you find out.

Sites with Helpful Information

www.diabetes.org

This is the website of the American Diabetes Association. It offers educational materials, including introductory information about diabetes, tips for weight loss and exercise, and diabetes-friendly recipes. There is also an online store where you can purchase books and other materials. The website has links to its message boards, which I think can be helpful. If you feel more comfortable over the telephone, you can call the American Diabetes Association at 1-800-DIABETES.

www.eatright.org

The website of the American Dietetic Association. While this site doesn't offer much for people with diabetes, it does contain some tips on eating healthy. It can also help you find a registered dietitian in your area.

www.niddk.nih.gov

This is the website for the National Institute of Diabetes and Digestive and Kidney Diseases, a part of the National Institutes of Health. All of the information on this government site is free, and it can be helpful if you just want the cold, hard facts on type 2 diabetes in America.

www.drbuynak.com

My personal website. It contains additional information about diabetes and diet as well as other useful links.

www.mypyramid.gov

The U.S. Department of Agriculture has formed a website dedicated to its new food pyramid. This website is very interactive and will help you plan your exercise and diet around healthy eating. It also offers some good feedback on your meal plan. The site does require patience and a healthy knowledge of computers and the Internet, so if you're really computer savvy, this might be your perfect resource. Nonetheless, this is a worthwhile place to visit.

Diet Systems

I'm not personally recommending any of these diet systems and neither am I discouraging you from viewing their websites. It's just that they will cost you money, and I think you can do this on your own at a lot less cost. But if you find that having a more directed meal plan provided by someone else will work better, go ahead and visit these sites.

www.seattlesutton.com

Seattle Sutton is a meal delivery system. Food is delivered to your home.

www.zonedietathome.com

The Zone Diet is another popular meal delivery system, much like Seattle Sutton.

www.weightwatchers.com

Weight Watchers is the famous point system for weight loss and is extremely popular. Many people swear by this method, which gives it a lot of credibility.

www.jennycraig.com

You've probably also heard of Jenny Craig, which is another weight-loss program. Jenny Craig provides consultations with registered dietitians, encourages and motivates healthy eating and exercise, and features a full meal plan and sells you special meals for the program.

BOOKS

General Diabetes Information

These popular and informative books provide general reference information in plain language for the person with diabetes. All of them are available through the American Diabetes Association.

American Diabetes Association Complete Guide to Diabetes, 4th edition, by the ADA.

Diabetes A to Z, by the ADA.

Type 2 Diabetes for Beginners, by Phyllis Barrier, MS, RD, CDE.

Cookbooks and Meal Planners

The cookbooks published by the American Diabetes Association are really helpful for people with diabetes because they always provide the nutritional information for the recipes. If you use exchange lists, these cookbooks also contain exchange values for each menu item. Some of these cookbooks even provide meal plans and tips on creating your own meal plans. The meal planners give tons of information on the nutritional content of foods you'll find in restaurants and in grocery stores. Some of them also have step-by-step instructions for creating your own meal plans.

Diabetes & Heart Healthy Cookbook, by the ADA and American Heart Association.

Month of Meals cookbook series. This series consists of several cookbooks, each featuring a different style of cooking. They're flip-books, so you can mix and match different recipes for each meal and ensure a balanced, healthy daily meal plan but still enjoy diverse foods. These must-buy cookbooks should be in the kitchen of everyone with diabetes.

Diabetes Meal Planning Made Easy, 2nd Edition, by Hope Warshaw, MMSc, RD, CDE, BC-ADM.

Complete Guide to Carb Counting, 2nd Edition, by Hope Warshaw, MMSc, RD, CDE, BC-ADM, and Karmeen Kulkarni, MS, RD, CDE, BC-ADM.

Diabetes Carbohydrate and Fat Gram Guide, 3rd Edition, by Lea Ann Holzmeister, RD, CDE.

The Diabetes Food and Nutrition Bible, by Hope Warshaw, MMSc, RD, CDE, BC-ADM, and Robyn Webb.

Guide to Healthy Restaurant Eating, 3rd edition, by Hope Warshaw, MMSc, RD, CDE, BC-ADM.

Exercise and Weight Loss

Small Steps, Big Rewards (book and pedometer package). This handy little kit is extremely helpful in getting started on physical activity. It includes a pedometer, which is a little device that counts how many steps you take when you wear it, and a book describing how to start walking for exercise. I highly recommend this item.

The "I Hate to Exercise" Book for People with Diabetes, by Charlotte Hayes, MMSc, MS, RD, CDE.

Complete Weight Loss Workbook, by Judith Wylie-Rosett, EdD, RD, Charles Swencionis, PhD, Arlene Caban, BS, Allison J. Friedler, BS, and Nicole Schaffer, MA.

Index

C

G

O

Other Titles Available from the American Diabetes Association

Guide to Healthy Restaurant Eating
By Hope S. Warshaw, MMSc, RD, CDE, BC-ADM
Eat out without guilt or sacrifice! Newly updated, this bestselling guide features more than 5,000 menu items for over 60 restaurant chains. This is the most comprehensive guide to restaurant nutrition for people with diabetes who like to eat out.
Order #4819-03
$17.95 US

Type 2 Diabetes for Beginners
By Phyllis Barrier, MS, RD, CDE
If you've recently been diagnosed with type 2 diabetes, this book is the introduction you need for staying healthy. You'll get the straight facts about living with type 2 diabetes and straight answers to your questions about the disease.
Order #4877-01
$14.95 US

The Diabetes Carbohydrate & Fat Gram Guide, 3rd Edition
By Lea Ann Holzmeister, RD, CDE
This guide is now better than ever. Registered dietitian Lea Ann Holzmeister has gone back to the drawing board and put together complete nutritional information, including carbs, fat, calories, and more for nearly 7,000 listings. This new edition now features charts for fast foods and prepackaged meals.
Order #4708-03
$14.95 US

American Diabetes Association Complete Guide to Diabetes, 4th Edition
By the American Diabetes Association
The world's largest collection of diabetes self-care tips, techniques, and tricks you can use to solve diabetes-related troubles just got bigger and better!
Order #4809-04
$29.95 US

To order these and other great American Diabetes Association titles, call 1-800-232-6733 or visit http://store.diabetes.org.
American Diabetes Association titles are also available in bookstores nationwide.

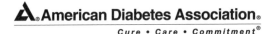
American Diabetes Association®
Cure • Care • Commitment®

About the
American Diabetes Association

The American Diabetes Association is the nation's leading voluntary health organization supporting diabetes research, information, and advocacy. Its mission is to prevent and cure diabetes and to improve the lives of all people affected by diabetes. The American Diabetes Association is the leading publisher of comprehensive diabetes information. Its huge library of practical and authoritative books for people with diabetes covers every aspect of self-care—cooking and nutrition, fitness, weight control, medications, complications, emotional issues, and general self-care.

To order American Diabetes Association books: Call 1-800-232-6733 or log on to http://store.diabetes.org

To join the American Diabetes Association: Call 1-800-806-7801 or log on to www.diabetes.org/membership

For more information about diabetes or ADA programs and services: Call 1-800-342-2383. E-mail: AskADA@diabetes.org or log on to www.diabetes.org

To locate an ADA/NCQA Recognized Provider of quality diabetes care in your area: www.ncqa.org/dprp

To find an ADA Recognized Education Program in your area: Call 1-800-342-2383. www.diabetes.org/for-health-professionals-and-scientists/recognition/edrecognition.jsp

To join the fight to increase funding for diabetes research, end discrimination, and improve insurance coverage: Call 1-800-342-2383. www.diabetes.org/advocacy-and-legalresources/advocacy.jsp

To find out how you can get involved with the programs in your community: Call 1-800-342-2383. See below for program Web addresses.

American Diabetes Month: educational activities aimed at those diagnosed with diabetes—month of November. www.diabetes.org/communityprograms-and-localevents/americandiabetesmonth.jsp

American Diabetes Alert: annual public awareness campaign to find the undiagnosed—held the fourth Tuesday in March. www.diabetes.org/communityprograms-and-localevents/americandiabetesalert.jsp

The Diabetes Assistance & Resources Program (DAR): diabetes awareness program targeted to the Latino community. www.diabetes.org/communityprograms-and-localevents/latinos.jsp

African American Program: diabetes awareness program targeted to the African American community. www.diabetes.org/communityprograms-and-localevents/africanamericans.jsp

Awakening the Spirit: Pathways to Diabetes Prevention & Control: diabetes awareness program targeted to the Native American community. www.diabetes.org/communityprograms-and-localevents/nativeamericans.jsp

To find out about an important research project regarding type 2 diabetes: www.diabetes.org/diabetes-research/research-home.jsp

To obtain information on making a planned gift or charitable bequest: Call 1-888-700-7029. www.wpg.cc/stl/CDA/homepage/1,1006,509,00.html

To make a donation or memorial contribution: Call 1-800-342-2383. www.diabetes.org/support-the-cause/make-a-donation.jsp